PREVENTING TRANSMISSION OF PANDEMIC INFLUENZA AND OTHER VIRAL RESPIRATORY DISEASES

Personal Protective Equipment for Healthcare Personnel

UPDATE 2010

Committee on Personal Protective Equipment for Healthcare Personnel to Prevent Transmission of Pandemic Influenza and Other Viral Respiratory Infections: Current Research Issues

Board on Health Sciences Policy

Elaine L. Larson and Catharyn T. Liverman, *Editors*

INSTITUTE OF MEDICINE
OF THE NATIONAL ACADEMIES

THE NATIONAL ACADEMIES PRESS
Washington, D.C.
www.nap.edu

THE NATIONAL ACADEMIES PRESS • 500 Fifth Street, N.W. • Washington, DC 20001

NOTICE: The project that is the subject of this report was approved by the Governing Board of the National Research Council, whose members are drawn from the councils of the National Academy of Sciences, the National Academy of Engineering, and the Institute of Medicine.

This study was requested by the National Institute for Occupational Safety and Health of the Centers for Disease Control and Prevention and was supported by Contract No. 200-2005-10881 (Task Order #8) between the National Academy of Sciences and the Centers for Disease Control and Prevention. Any opinions, findings, conclusions, or recommendations expressed in this publication are those of the author(s) and do not necessarily reflect the view of the organizations or agencies that provided support for this project.

International Standard Book Number-13: 978-0-309-16254-8
International Standard Book Number-10: 0-309-16254-8

Additional copies of this report are available from the National Academies Press, 500 Fifth Street, N.W., Lockbox 285, Washington, DC 20055; (800) 624-6242 or (202) 334-3313 (in the Washington metropolitan area); Internet, http://www.nap.edu.

For more information about the Institute of Medicine, visit the IOM home page at: **www.iom.edu.**

The serpent has been a symbol of long life, healing, and knowledge among almost all cultures and religions since the beginning of recorded history. The serpent adopted as a logotype by the Institute of Medicine is a relief carving from ancient Greece, now held by the Staatliche Museen in Berlin.

Suggested citation: IOM (Institute of Medicine). 2011. *Preventing transmission of pandemic influenza and other viral respiratory diseases: Personal protective equipment for healthcare personnel. Update 2010.* Washington, DC: The National Academies Press.

"Knowing is not enough; we must apply.
Willing is not enough; we must do."
—Goethe

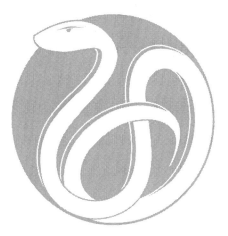

INSTITUTE OF MEDICINE
OF THE NATIONAL ACADEMIES

Advising the Nation. Improving Health.

THE NATIONAL ACADEMIES
Advisers to the Nation on Science, Engineering, and Medicine

The **National Academy of Sciences** is a private, nonprofit, self-perpetuating society of distinguished scholars engaged in scientific and engineering research, dedicated to the furtherance of science and technology and to their use for the general welfare. Upon the authority of the charter granted to it by the Congress in 1863, the Academy has a mandate that requires it to advise the federal government on scientific and technical matters. Dr. Ralph J. Cicerone is president of the National Academy of Sciences.

The **National Academy of Engineering** was established in 1964, under the charter of the National Academy of Sciences, as a parallel organization of outstanding engineers. It is autonomous in its administration and in the selection of its members, sharing with the National Academy of Sciences the responsibility for advising the federal government. The National Academy of Engineering also sponsors engineering programs aimed at meeting national needs, encourages education and research, and recognizes the superior achievements of engineers. Dr. Charles M. Vest is president of the National Academy of Engineering.

The **Institute of Medicine** was established in 1970 by the National Academy of Sciences to secure the services of eminent members of appropriate professions in the examination of policy matters pertaining to the health of the public. The Institute acts under the responsibility given to the National Academy of Sciences by its congressional charter to be an adviser to the federal government and, upon its own initiative, to identify issues of medical care, research, and education. Dr. Harvey V. Fineberg is president of the Institute of Medicine.

The **National Research Council** was organized by the National Academy of Sciences in 1916 to associate the broad community of science and technology with the Academy's purposes of furthering knowledge and advising the federal government. Functioning in accordance with general policies determined by the Academy, the Council has become the principal operating agency of both the National Academy of Sciences and the National Academy of Engineering in providing services to the government, the public, and the scientific and engineering communities. The Council is administered jointly by both Academies and the Institute of Medicine. Dr. Ralph J. Cicerone and Dr. Charles M. Vest are chair and vice chair, respectively, of the National Research Council.

www.national-academies.org

Study Staff

CATHARYN T. LIVERMAN, Project Director
ANDREW M. POPE, Director
SARAH CODREA, Associate Program Officer (until July 2010)
LARA ANDERSEN, Research Associate
JUDY ESTEP, Program Associate

Reviewers

This report has been reviewed in draft form by individuals chosen for their diverse perspectives and technical expertise, in accordance with procedures approved by the National Research Council's Report Review Committee. The purpose of this independent review is to provide candid and critical comments that will assist the institution in making its published report as sound as possible and to ensure that the report meets institutional standards for objectivity, evidence, and responsiveness to the study charge. The review comments and draft manuscript remain confidential to protect the integrity of the deliberative process. We wish to thank the following individuals for their review of this report:

Lisa Brosseau, University of Minnesota
Benjamin Cowling, University of Hong Kong
Lewis R. Goldfrank, Bellevue Hospital Center and New York
    University Medical Center
Kathleen Harriman, California Department of Public Health
Sundaresan Jayaraman, Georgia Institute of Technology
Mark Nicas, University of California
Daniel R. Perez, University of Maryland
Trish M. Perl, Johns Hopkins University School of Medicine
Peg Seminario, AFL–CIO
Michael Tapper, Lenox Hill Hospital, New York City
David Weber, University of North Carolina–Chapel Hill
Annalee Yassi, University of British Columbia

Although the reviewers listed above have provided many constructive comments and suggestions, they were not asked to endorse the conclusions or recommendations, nor did they see the final draft of the report before its release. The review of this report was overseen by **Caroline Breese Hall,** University of Rochester School of Medicine, and **Johanna T. Dwyer,** Tufts University School of Medicine. Appointed by the National Research Council and Institute of Medicine, they were responsible for making certain that an independent examination of this report was carried out in accordance with institutional procedures and that all review comments were carefully considered. Responsibility for the final content of this report rests entirely with the authoring committee and the institution.

Contents

Acronyms and Abbreviations

AAMI	Association for the Advancement of Medical Instrumentation
B.R.E.A.T.H.E.	Better Respiratory Equipment Using Advanced Technologies for Healthcare Employees
CBRN	chemical, biological, radiological, and nuclear
CDC	Centers for Disease Control and Prevention
CFR	Code of Federal Regulations
CI	confidence interval
CO_2	carbon dioxide
DOL	Department of Labor
FDA	Food and Drug Administration
FFP2 or FFP3	filtering facepiece respirator class P2 or P3
HHS	Department of Health and Human Services
ICU	intensive care unit
IOM	Institute of Medicine
IV	intravenous
MPPS	most penetrating particle size
NaCl	sodium chloride
NIOSH	National Institute for Occupational Safety and Health

NPPTL	National Personal Protective Technology Laboratory
NVHA	Northern Virginia Hospital Alliance
NYC	New York City
OSHA	Occupational Safety and Health Administration
PAPR	powered air-purifying respirator
PPE	personal protective equipment
PPT	personal protective technologies
RNA	ribonucleic acid
RSV	respiratory syncytial virus
RT-PCR	real-time polymerase chain reaction
SARS	severe acute respiratory syndrome
SNS	Strategic National Stockpile
$TICD_{50}$	tissue culture infective dose$_{50}$
TIL	total inward leakage
UV	ultraviolet
WHO	World Health Organization

Summary

In 2008, the Institute of Medicine (IOM) published the report *Preparing for an Influenza Pandemic: Personal Protective Equipment for Healthcare Workers*. At the time of that report, the major influenza-related concern was avian influenza (H5N1). As novel H1N1 influenza A became a reality in 2009, the many unknowns about the virulence, spread, and nature of the virus raised to the forefront issues regarding personal protective equipment (PPE) for healthcare personnel. A major issue was the nature of respiratory protection required because much remains to be learned about the mechanisms of influenza transmission. This report comes at a time when controversies continue on issues related to PPE for healthcare personnel, while at the same time, new horizons in PPE research and attention to PPE innovations offer promise of improvements in healthcare worker safety. Keeping the research momentum going is critical, because between pandemics the focus of research efforts often moves to other issues and the nation remains underprepared.

SCOPE OF THE REPORT

The 2009–2010 H1N1 experience and its accompanying unanswered research questions provided the impetus for the National Personal Protective Technology Laboratory (NPPTL) at the National Institute for Occupational Safety and Health (NIOSH) to ask the IOM to conduct a study that would update progress on research and identify future directions regarding PPE for healthcare personnel.[1]

This report is the result of a 12-month study conducted by an ad hoc IOM committee composed of experts in the fields of infectious disease, infection control, public health, occupational safety and health, pulmonary medicine, health promotion, microbiology, emergency response and preparedness, epidemiology, nursing, community health, industrial hygiene, and materials engineering. The IOM committee was charged with identifying new research directions, certification[2] and standards-setting issues, and risk assessment issues specific to PPE for healthcare personnel to prevent transmission of pandemic influenza and other viral respiratory infections. The committee was specifically asked to focus on the following issues:

- research needed to understand and improve the efficacy and effectiveness of PPE, particularly face masks and respirators, for preventing transmission of pandemic influenza or other viral respiratory infections. Specific attention was sought on issues related to the research needed to determine the type of respiratory protection needed for the given exposure, to determine the requirements for protective ensembles to provide an appropriate level of protection based on work tasks, and to improve functionality and address human factor issues such as wearability, compliance, and communications;
- necessary certification, testing, and standards development issues; and
- priorities and resources for research and certification efforts.

To accomplish its charge, the committee held three meetings and gathered information through a scientific workshop that included a public comment session, through discussions with numerous individuals in the infection control and occupational safety and health fields, and through a review of the relevant literature. As mentioned above, this report builds on the work of the IOM committee that released the 2008 report, and

---

[1] The committee broadly defines "healthcare personnel" to encompass all workers in direct patient care and support services who are employed by private and public healthcare offices and facilities as well as those working in home health care and emergency medical services, including those who are self-employed.

[2] The committee broadly defines "certification" to encompass the entire conformity assessment process.

throughout this report, the prior work is summarized. In large part, this committee's task was to examine research conducted since the 2008 report, to assess where research stands on issues key to improving PPE for healthcare personnel exposed to infectious respiratory diseases, and to make recommendations to address current research gaps. Many PPE issues relevant to healthcare personnel are also directly relevant to the PPE needs of workers in other occupations, as well as the general public.

PPE FOR HEALTHCARE PERSONNEL

The term "personal protective equipment" encompasses the specialized clothing or equipment worn by workers for protection against health and safety hazards. For healthcare personnel, PPE may include respirators, face masks, gloves,[3] eye protection, face shields, gowns, and head and shoe coverings. Integrating the various types of protective equipment to ensure that they work together as ensembles (e.g., eye protection with a respirator) is an ongoing concern. Infection prevention and control in healthcare workplaces involve, among many other measures, the use of PPE. Infection control precautions follow a tiered approach that considers the possible routes of transmission among patients and healthcare personnel.

One of the challenges for the healthcare field is to clearly understand the differences between respirators and face masks as well as their appropriate uses. Respirators are specifically designed as respiratory protection. They work either by purifying the air inhaled by the wearer through filtering materials or by independently supplying breathable air. For air-purifying respirators (often the type used by healthcare personnel) the major issues are the filtration and the fit—the effectiveness of the filter and the extent to which the respirator has a tight seal with the wearer's face to restrict inward leakage.

Face masks, including surgical masks and procedure masks, are loose-fitting coverings that are designed to protect the patient from secretions from the nose and mouth of the physician, nurse, or other healthcare professional. Face masks are not designed or certified to protect the wearer from exposure to respiratory hazards; the role of face masks as PPE requires further research.

---

[3]Hand hygiene is another important and effective component of infection control of respiratory diseases, but is not within the scope of this report.

Measures to prevent influenza transmission to healthcare personnel include all levels of hazard controls. PPE along with vaccination and antiviral medications are components of an overall infection prevention and control program that uses engineering, administrative, and work practice controls. Although all levels of this hierarchy are important, this report is focused on opportunities to improve PPE and the correct use of PPE in healthcare settings.

In discussing the issues relevant to the use of PPE by healthcare personnel, the committee identified a set of criteria as a starting point for decisions on PPE selection and use. PPE for healthcare personnel should

- effectively reduce risks of disease or injury to healthcare personnel;
- minimize negative interactions with or effects on patients, their families, and caregivers;
- be acceptable and usable by healthcare personnel in their daily tasks, including ease of communication and comfort;
- be practical regarding issues of cost, time, and training; and
- be appropriate to the occupational risk being encountered.

Having recently been through the 2009–2010 experience with H1N1 influenza, the committee is well aware of the ongoing challenges and controversies surrounding PPE for healthcare personnel. At this time, it is particularly important to build on that experience and take the actions needed to address the research and policy questions that will allow the healthcare community to be better prepared for the next epidemic or pandemic. Experience has shown that relevant research on these issues wanes between pandemics, and not permitting that to happen this time is crucial to resolving the research questions and setting evidence-based policies in place.

UPDATE ON PROGRESS: 2007 TO 2010

Transmission of Influenza and Other Viral Respiratory Diseases

Animal studies have found that the ferret and guinea pig models appear to be highly representative of humans in terms of their susceptibility to infection, the influenza viral strains that display a transmissible phenotype, and the kinetics with which transmission occurs. Experiments performed in both of these animal models suggest that transmission of influenza viruses can proceed by both droplet spray and aerosol routes, which would include respirable particles. Animal studies have also pointed to a number of environmental factors, including relative humidity and temperature, that may influence transmission. Recent studies that employed environmental monitoring of air for influenza as well as others that examined the contamination of fomites and hands with H1N1 have provided insights on the potential for influenza virus contamination of the healthcare environment. Nonetheless, data on the viability of influenza and other respiratory viruses in air samples and on fomites in these settings are limited. Mathematical models have been developed to better characterize the relative contribution of influenza transmission modes. Available, well-specified parameters for these models are limited because information is lacking on the viability of influenza in aerosols, salivary virus concentrations, the amount of virus in respirable and inspirable particles, and the quantity and persistence of viability on various fomites in the healthcare setting. Taken together, progress has been made in understanding the modes of transmission, but the relative contribution of the modes are still unclear. Much remains to be learned about the effectiveness of control measures to prevent transmission.

Observational and controlled studies relevant to PPE use and transmission of influenza or other viral respiratory diseases are limited because study protocols were not usually in place for 2009 H1N1 or for recent seasonal flu periods, and studies have not provided adequate power to answer questions regarding the effectiveness of using PPE in reducing or preventing disease transmission.

Designing and Engineering Effective PPE

PPE is a critical component in the hierarchy of controls used to protect healthcare personnel from influenza and other viral respiratory diseases. Understanding the functional issues related to the design of PPE, as well as the factors that impact use, is critical to ensuring that healthcare personnel are adequately protected and comfortable and can perform their jobs. Important advances have been made in some areas since the last report, but other areas, particularly regarding improvements in gowns, gloves, face masks, and face shields, need to be more fully addressed. Much research has been done regarding filtration of respirator media, but ways to improve fit, including new technologies specifically for filtering facepiece respirators, need more research because face seal leakage greatly exceeds filter penetration in the overall total inward leakage of respirators. The physiological impact of respirators has been studied in depth, but research in this area is lacking regarding other types of PPE. Integration issues concerning PPE and medical equipment and the impact on operational performance have not been adequately studied. Effective decontamination methods that do not impact the physical characteristics of respirators have been studied for some types of respirators, but with inconclusive results. Finally, the characteristics of a respirator that would specifically address the needs of healthcare personnel (e.g., patient–provider interaction, comfort, reduced physiological burden) have been identified. Addressing these issues is important for developing PPE for healthcare personnel that is safe, effective, and comfortable.

Using PPE: Individual and Organizational Issues

Research during the past several years reveals modest gains in understanding that self-protective behavior in the healthcare settings involves a constellation of interacting and independent components. At a minimum, consideration should be given to the user, the device, the task, and the general work and organizational context. The growing acknowledgment of contextual and organizational factors means that research on PPE and healthcare personnel is closing in on the larger body of occupational safety research, which increasingly emphasizes those factors in understanding occupational safety performance.

Although there are clear gaps and deficiencies in our knowledge base about PPE usage in health care, existing knowledge is sufficient to recommend a four-pronged strategy for immediate implementation. The four elements are: (1) deliberate planning and preparation at the leadership and organizational levels; (2) comprehensive training, including supervisors and managers; (3) widespread and convenient availability of appropriate PPE devices; and (4) accountability at all levels of the organization.

In essence, there should be universal acknowledgement that PPE use is an integral component of providing quality health care. As with other priorities, this aspect of healthcare delivery needs to be carefully planned at the organizational/institutional level. Furthermore, managers and frontline workers alike need to understand and accept their roles and responsibilities, and PPE use needs to be as easy and convenient as possible. PPE should be factored into all decisions involving task design, staffing, and work assignments. Input from frontline workers should be used to facilitate planning and decision making and to maximize acceptance. Environmental/engineering controls should be utilized wherever possible to control exposures, with PPE used as a supplement or alternative when environmental/engineering controls are not sufficient or feasible. The overall implementation of the PPE program should be monitored regularly, with the goals of continuous improvement, adoption of best practices, and accountability of both supervisor and worker.

Policy Research and Implementation

Preparations and implementation of infection control plans for 2009 H1N1 influenza brought into sharp focus the efforts by healthcare professionals, emergency planners, professional associations, healthcare facilities, policy makers, government agencies, labor unions, and others to address PPE policies and logistics. Articles continue to be published on the recent experience and the challenges and successes in providing face masks, respirators, and other PPE to healthcare personnel. As lessons learned during that experience continue to add to the body of knowledge, incorporating this information into research, policy, and practice efforts will be important. In the initial phases of an epidemic or pandemic—when there are many unknowns about the virus or agent—one of the challenges is to determine PPE policy and then to adapt those policies as information is gained on the severity, transmission, and nature of the disease, with an emphasis on communicating the changes. Standards-setting, regulatory, training, and research efforts continue to move toward improved respiratory protection, and recent work has begun to focus on the specifics of how to tailor PPE devices and PPE training to address the specific needs of healthcare personnel.

RECOMMENDATIONS: A SYSTEMS APPROACH TO PPE RESEARCH

Providing care to ill or injured patients involves a range of potentially hazardous exposures for healthcare personnel. Current infection control precautions address this challenge by providing guidance on PPE and other precautions that varies depending on the mode of transmission of the pathogen. The ultimate goal would be to have the definitive information that would match the appropriate type of PPE with the pathogen, its mode of transmission, the infectious dose, and its risk to healthcare personnel. In many cases in industrial settings, this level of specificity is available for chemical exposures, although other industrial settings with unknown or mixed exposures continue to pose challenges. Reaching that point for protecting healthcare personnel will require concerted research efforts.

This report explores an integrated approach that addresses the full spectrum of research (from basic research to policy research) and translates research findings into improvements in the standards of healthcare practice (Figure S-1). This approach ensures that basic science initiatives are fully explored while also addressing clinical needs and testing the results in real-world settings, with the expectation that adaptations along the way will be made and tested. Feedback loops to prior stages are also critically important. Such an integrated approach calls for active collaboration and discourse among scientists and clinicians who may not have had previous interactions.

Throughout this report, the committee has highlighted a number of areas in which research is needed. This research has the potential to quickly translate new understandings of disease transmission or PPE engineering into more effective PPE products. Fully implementing these research directions and realizing breakthroughs for improved safety and health for healthcare personnel will require commitments from multiple

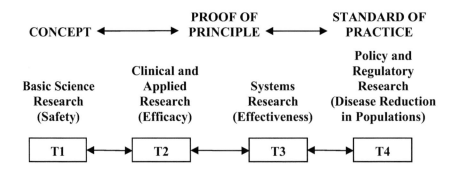

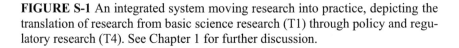

FIGURE S-1 An integrated system moving research into practice, depicting the translation of research from basic science research (T1) through policy and regulatory research (T4). See Chapter 1 for further discussion.

federal agencies as well as ongoing, innovative efforts by PPE designers and manufacturers. The report makes the following recommendations to advance research and transfer these into practice across the spectrum of research opportunities.

Across the Spectrum of Research

Recommendation: <u>Develop Standardized Terms and Definitions</u>
The Centers for Disease Control and Prevention (CDC) and the Occupational Safety and Health Administration (OSHA), in partnership with other relevant agencies and organizations, should work to develop standardized terms, definitions, and appropriate classifications to describe transmission routes and aerodynamic diameter of particles associated with respiratory disease transmission. This effort should involve a consensus from the industrial hygiene, infectious disease, and healthcare communities.

Recommendation: <u>Develop and Implement a Comprehensive Research Strategy to Understand Viral Respiratory Disease Transmission</u>
The National Institutes of Health, in collaboration with other research agencies and organizations, should develop and fund a comprehensive research strategy to improve the understanding of viral respiratory disease transmission, including, but not limited to, examining the characteristics of influenza transmission, animal models, human challenge studies, and intervention trials. This strategy should include

- **an expedited mechanism for funding these types of studies and**
- **clinical research centers of excellence for studying influenza and other respiratory virus transmission.**

Safety to Efficacy:
Basic Science Research (T1) to Clinical and Applied Research (T2)

Recommendation: Continue and Expand Research on PPE for Healthcare Personnel
NPPTL and other agencies, private-sector companies, and other organizations should continue to advance research in designing and evaluating the effectiveness of respirator protection for healthcare personnel and expand its research efforts to improve and evaluate the effectiveness of gloves, gowns, eye protection, face shields, and face masks in preventing the transmission of influenza or other viral respiratory diseases. Areas of focused research needs include

- effectiveness in preventing fomite, droplet spray, or aerosol transmission;
- decontamination and reusability;
- comfort, fit, and usability;
- impact on task performance; and
- development of technologies specifically for healthcare personnel.

Recommendation: Examine the Effectiveness of Face Masks and Face Shields as PPE
NPPTL should investigate the effectiveness of face masks and face shields in preventing transmission of viral respiratory diseases.

Recommendation: Improve Fit Test Methods and Evaluate User Seal Checks
NPPTL should develop novel, simpler fit test methods and evaluate the effectiveness of performing user seal checks on N95 respirators.

Efficacy to Effectiveness:
Clinical and Applied Research (T2) to Systems Research (T3)

Recommendation: Explore Healthcare Safety Culture and Work Organization

NIOSH and other relevant agencies, such as the Agency for Healthcare Research and Quality, and professional organizations should conduct research to better understand the role of safety culture and other behavioral and organizational factors on PPE usage in healthcare settings. These efforts should include

- conducting human factors and ergonomics research relevant to the design and organization of healthcare work tasks to improve worker safety by reducing hazardous exposures and effectively using PPE (e.g., reduce unnecessary PPE donning and doffing),
- exploring the links between patient safety and healthcare worker safety and health that are relevant to the use of PPE, and
- identifying and evaluating strategies to mitigate organizational barriers that limit the use of PPE by healthcare personnel.

Recommendation: <u>Identify and Disseminate Effective Leadership and Training Strategies and Other Interventions to Improve PPE Use</u>
NIOSH and other relevant agencies and professional organizations should support intervention effectiveness research to assess strategies, including innovative participatory approaches to training, for healthcare and supervisory staff at all levels to improve PPE usage and other related outcomes across the range of healthcare settings. To identify best practices, efforts should be made to

- conduct observational studies of PPE use by healthcare personnel in different types of work settings;
- develop, implement, and evaluate comprehensive leadership and training strategies and interventions that go beyond simple knowledge-based training;
- design training interventions specifically for supervisory and managerial personnel in different types of healthcare settings;
- examine long-term practice change and safety culture implementation related to educational interventions;

- improve use and understanding of PPE by home and community healthcare personnel;
- develop assessment tools and metrics that take a broader approach to PPE and acknowledge the interaction of worker, task, and environmental factors; and
- be informed by a lessons-learned summit on PPE use by healthcare personnel during the 2009 H1N1 experience.

Effectiveness to Disease Reduction in Populations: Systems Research (T3) to Policy and Regulatory Research (T4)

Recommendation: Develop and Certify Powered Air-Purifying Respirators (PAPRs) for Healthcare Personnel
NPPTL should develop certification requirements for a low-noise, loose-fitting PAPR for healthcare personnel.

Recommendation: Move Forward on Better Fitting Respirators
NPPTL should continue rulemaking processes for total inward leakage regulations that require respirators to meet fit criteria. To improve consumer and purchaser information on fit capabilities, NIOSH should establish a website to disseminate fit test results for specific respirator models on an anthropometric (NIOSH) test panel, where such data exist.

Recommendation: Clarify PPE Guidelines for Outbreaks of Novel Viral Respiratory Infections
NIOSH, other divisions of CDC, OSHA, and other public health agencies should develop a coordinated process to make, announce, and revise consistent guidelines regarding the use of PPE to be worn by healthcare personnel during a verified sustained national/international outbreak of a novel viral respiratory infection. The agencies should tailor their guidance in a timely and coordinated manner as the virulence, contagiousness, and affected populations are further characterized.

Recommendation: <u>Standards and Certification for Face Masks and Face Shields</u>
NIOSH, OSHA, and standards-development organizations should develop the standards and certification processes needed to assess the performance of face masks and face shields as PPE. The development of standards and certification processes should be guided by research regarding their efficacy as PPE:

- OSHA and CDC should clarify that face masks are governed by the general PPE standard (29 CFR 1910.132) and not by the respiratory protection standard (29 CFR 1910.134).
- NIOSH should work with other agencies and standards-setting organizations to develop voluntary consensus standards and independent third-party testing and certification processes for face shields and face masks with specific tests for assessing prevention of transmission of viral respiratory diseases.

Recommendation: <u>Establish PPE Regulations for Healthcare Personnel</u>
CDC, including NIOSH, and OSHA should develop and promulgate guidelines and regulations that are consistent regarding the use of PPE by healthcare personnel for influenza and other viral respiratory diseases:

- To assist employers in complying with the OSHA PPE standard, OSHA should specify the voluntary consensus standards that are required to be met for non-respirator PPE (e.g., gowns, gloves, face shields, face masks) in the event of influenza and other viral respiratory diseases.
- OSHA, with input from CDC and other agencies and organizations, should work toward promulgating an aerosol-transmissible diseases standard that would include prevention of the transmission of influenza and other viral respiratory diseases.

While the optimist can seek comfort in the fact that progress has been made in the past several years, the pragmatist must wonder about the rate of progress (or lack thereof) on such a critical issue that potentially threatens the security and economic well-being of the nation and the world. The committee hopes that this review will jumpstart and strengthen improvements in PPE for healthcare personnel that could be relevant to a range of viral respiratory diseases.

1

Introduction

In 2008, the Institute of Medicine (IOM) published the report *Preparing for an Influenza Pandemic: Personal Protective Equipment for Healthcare Workers* (IOM, 2008). When the report was released, the major influenza-related concern was avian influenza (H5N1). As novel H1N1 influenza A became a reality in 2009, the many unknowns about the virulence, spread, and nature of the virus raised to the forefront issues regarding personal protective equipment (PPE) for healthcare personnel. One of the major issues was the nature of respiratory protection required because much remains to be learned about the mechanisms of influenza transmission. This current report comes at a time when controversies continue on issues related to PPE for healthcare personnel while new horizons in PPE research and attention to PPE innovations offer promise for improvements in healthcare worker safety. Keeping the research momentum moving forward is critical, because between pandemics the focus of research efforts often moves to other issues and the nation remains underprepared.

SCOPE OF THE REPORT

The 2009–2010 H1N1 experience and its accompanying unanswered research questions provided the impetus for the National Personal Protective Technology Laboratory (NPPTL) at the National Institute for Occupational Safety and Health (NIOSH) to ask the IOM to conduct a study that would update the progress on research and identify future directions regarding PPE use for healthcare personnel.

This report is the result of a 12-month study conducted by an ad hoc IOM committee composed of experts in the fields of infectious disease, infection control, public health, occupational safety and health, pulmonary medicine, health promotion, microbiology, emergency preparedness and response, epidemiology, nursing, community health, industrial hygiene, and materials engineering. The IOM committee was charged with identifying new research directions, certification[1] and standards-setting issues, and risk assessment issues specific to PPE for healthcare personnel to prevent transmission of pandemic influenza and other viral respiratory infections. The committee was asked to focus specifically on the following areas:

- research needed to understand and improve the efficacy and effectiveness of personal protective equipment, particularly face masks and respirators for preventing transmission of pandemic influenza or other viral respiratory infections. Specific attention was sought on issues related to the research needed to determine the type of respiratory protection needed for the given exposure, to determine the requirements for protective ensembles to provide an appropriate level of protection based on work tasks, and to improve functionality and address human factor issues, such as wearability, compliance, and communications;
- necessary certification, testing, and standards development issues; and
- priorities and resources for research and certification efforts.

To accomplish its charge, the committee held three meetings and gathered information through a scientific workshop (Appendix A) that included a public comment session, discussions with numerous individuals in the infection control and occupational safety and health fields, and a review of the relevant literature. As mentioned above, this report builds on the work of the IOM committee that released the 2008 report. Throughout this report, the prior work is summarized. In large part, this committee's task was to examine research conducted since the 2008 report in order to assess where research stands on issues that are key to improving PPE for healthcare personnel exposed to infectious respiratory diseases and to make recommendations to address current research gaps.

---

[1]The committee broadly defines "certification" to encompass the entire conformity assessment process.

Many PPE issues relevant to healthcare personnel are also directly relevant to the PPE needs of workers in other occupations as well as the general public.

In 2009, an Institute of Medicine committee addressed the question of what type of PPE was needed for the 2009 H1N1 pandemic. In addition to recommending the use of respirators because respiratory protection was deemed appropriate, the report recommended increased research on "the next generation of personal respiratory protection technologies for healthcare workers to enhance safety, comfort, and ability to perform work-related tasks" (IOM, 2009).

BACKGROUND AND CONTEXT

Readers of this report may be familiar with the 2008 report or knowledgeable about the extensive background issues regarding PPE and its use in healthcare settings. In lieu of including extensive background materials, the committee provides an overview of the context for this report by addressing the following series of questions.

What Are PPE and Personal Protective Technologies?

The term "personal protective equipment" encompasses the specialized clothing or equipment worn by workers for protection against health and safety hazards. Specific types of PPE are selected based on the occupational hazard faced in specific work tasks or sites. "Personal protective technologies" is a broader term that includes the protective equipment as well as the technical methods, processes, techniques, tools, and materials that support their development, evaluation, and use (NIOSH, 2007; OSHA, 2002). This report most often discusses the equipment used by healthcare personnel and uses the term "PPE," although in some cases the broader term is needed.

For healthcare personnel, PPE may include respirators, face masks, gloves,[2] eye protection, face shields, gowns, and head and shoe coverings. Respirators provide respiratory protection; the other products are designed primarily to provide a barrier against microbes contacting the skin or mucous membrane surfaces. Integrating the various types of pro-

---

[2]Hand hygiene is another important and effective component of infection control of respiratory diseases, but it is not within the purview of this report.

tective equipment to ensure that they work together as ensembles (e.g., eye protection with a respirator) is an ongoing concern. Infection prevention and control in healthcare workplaces involve, among many other measures, the use of PPE.

What Are the Roles of Face Masks and Respirators?

One of the challenges for the healthcare field is to clearly understand the differences between respirators and face masks as well as their appropriate uses. In this report, the terminology used by the investigators or authors of the cited journal article or report is used, but in some cases, determining whether the authors' use of the term "masks" refers to face masks, respirators, or both was impossible.

Face masks, including surgical and procedure masks, are loose-fitting coverings of the nose and mouth that are designed to protect the patient from secretions from the nose or mouth of the physician, nurse, or other healthcare professional. Face masks are not designed or certified to protect the wearer from exposure to respiratory hazards. Some studies have looked at the variation in filtration capabilities of face masks (Chapter 3), but the role of face masks as PPE requires further research.

Respirators are specifically designed as respiratory protection and are certified by NIOSH (42 Code of Federal Regulations [CFR] Part 84). They work either by purifying the air inhaled by the wearer through filtering materials or by independently supplying breathable air. For air-purifying respirators (often the type used by healthcare personnel), the major issues are the filtration and the fit—the effectiveness of the filter and the extent to which the respirator has a tight seal with the wearer's face to restrict inward leakage. A type of respirators, termed surgical N95 respirators, is cleared by the Food and Drug Administration (FDA) as medical devices. To be effective, respirators must fit tightly to the face. Annual fit testing for respirators is required by the Occupational Safety and Health Administration (OSHA), and user seal checks are required with each use (29 CFR 1910.134).

How Does PPE Fit into the Range of Other Workplace Safety and Preventive Measures?

Efforts to promote worker safety and health traditionally follow a hierarchy of controls. *Engineering and environmental measures*, such as air exchanges (including non-recirculated exchanges) or negative-pressure rooms that can isolate the hazard or reduce exposure, are ubiquitous measures that affect a large number of workers and patients and do not depend on individual compliance (IOM, 2008). *Administrative controls* are next in the hierarchy and include the policies, standards, procedures, and practices established within an organization to limit hazardous exposures and improve worker safety (e.g., vaccination policies, cohorting or isolating patients, hand hygiene measures, provision of appropriate and effective PPE, organizational commitment to creating and sustaining a culture of worker safety) (IOM, 2009). At the level of *work practice controls*, including *individual practices*, the healthcare employer and individual personnel are responsible for appropriate use of PPE as well as being vaccinated and adhering to work safety practices.

Measures to prevent transmission of influenza or other viral respiratory diseases to healthcare personnel include all levels of hazard controls. PPE, along with vaccination and antiviral medications, are components of an overall infection prevention and control program that uses engineering, administrative, and work practice controls. Vaccination against influenza has been found to be effective in preventing the illness in the recipient with overall efficacy rates over 70 percent (Fiore et al., 2009; Treanor et al., 1999).[3] Although all levels of this hierarchy are important, this report focuses on opportunities to improve PPE and the correct use of PPE in healthcare settings.

What Federal Agencies Are Involved in Healthcare Personnel PPE?

The testing, regulation, and use of PPE by healthcare personnel involve several federal departments and agencies. Responsibilities for occupational health and safety are within the purview of both the Department of Health and Human Services (HHS) and the Department of

---

[3]The Centers for Disease Control and Prevention has noted that the influenza vaccination coverage goal for healthcare personnel should be 100 percent of employees who do not have medical contraindications and that the level of vaccination coverage among healthcare personnel can serve as a measure of a patient safety quality program (CDC, 2010b).

Labor (DOL). The *Occupational Safety and Health Act of 1970* (Public Law 91-596) created two federal agencies that focus on worker safety and health: NIOSH (in HHS) is designated with responsibilities for relevant research, training, and education; and OSHA (in DOL) is designated with responsibilities for developing and enforcing workplace safety and health regulations.

NPPTL, a NIOSH laboratory, conducts and funds research on improvements in PPE and ensembles used in a variety of occupations. NPPTL also plays an integral role in standards-setting efforts relevant to PPE. Respirators used by personnel in OSHA-regulated workplaces, including healthcare workplaces, must be NIOSH certified. OSHA respirator regulations detail employer responsibilities for establishing and maintaining a comprehensive respiratory protection program, including selection, training, and fit testing requirements. For other types of PPE, OSHA specifies the voluntary consensus standards that the equipment must meet as well as relevant selection and training requirements. NIOSH, through NPPTL, conducts an extensive array of tests to assess respirator performance characteristics and to determine if the respirator meets the certification requirements.

To be marketed in the United States as medical devices, manufacturers of respirators, face masks, and some other types of healthcare PPE are required to obtain FDA approval or clearance by demonstrating equivalence with a similar product on the market. A number of other departments and agencies are involved in various aspects of healthcare PPE. In addition to NIOSH within the Centers for Disease Control and Prevention (CDC), the National Center for Emerging and Zoonotic Infectious Diseases, in conjunction with the external Healthcare Infection Control Practices Advisory Committee (HICPAC), develops infection control guidance for healthcare settings (CDC, 2010c). Public health agencies at the local, state, and federal levels play an instrumental role in developing guidelines, providing training, and assisting healthcare facilities with PPE-related issues. The Department of Defense and the Department of Veterans Affairs are actively involved in testing and developing PPE for military and veterans' care applications. The Department of Homeland Security focuses on emergency response PPE and works to coordinate and improve standards and equipment-related issues. The Environmental Protection Agency addresses PPE issues relevant to emergency response readiness. The Consumer Product Safety Commission has oversight responsibilities for products sold in the commercial marketplace, including

PPE.[4] Professional associations, standards development organizations, and other entities also play important roles in ensuring that PPE products meet performance criteria.

How Does This Report Define the Scope
of the Term "Healthcare Personnel"?

More than 14 million U.S. workers are employed in health care (BLS, 2010). The committee broadly defines "healthcare personnel" to encompass all workers in direct patient care and support services who are employed by private and public healthcare offices and facilities as well as those working in home healthcare and emergency medical services, including those who are self-employed. This broad definition of healthcare personnel encompasses those working in administration, patient care, and facilities upkeep, and it includes health professional students who are receiving instruction or who are working in healthcare facilities as well as volunteers trained to provide systematic, regulated, and licensed healthcare services (including emergency medical responders) (IOM, 2008, 2009). All relevant work situations with the potential for infection risk (e.g., cleaning patient rooms, delivering food) are considered part of the healthcare workforce. This definition is expanded from the definition used in the 2008 report. The committee acknowledges that, in the midst of an influenza pandemic, many people outside the traditional healthcare workforce will become caregivers, including many family members, and they may need access to PPE.

HEALTHCARE PERSONNEL AND PPE

Many work environments offer challenges for protecting personnel—the heat and smoke of firefighting, the heights of construction work on rooftops and high-rise buildings, and worksite noise or hazardous chemicals in industrial settings—to name a few. For healthcare personnel, several aspects of the job provide challenges for designing and wearing

---

[4]As noted in the 2008 report, PPE products that assert protection against a specific health hazard must have FDA approval or market clearance. Other PPE products sold in the commercial marketplace do not have requirements stipulating premarket or other testing prior to their sale to the public. For those products that assert NIOSH certification, NIOSH has the authority to act against mislabeled products.

appropriate PPE. These issues include interactions with patients and family members that make communication critically important, split-second actions in some healthcare situations that can have major consequences, and challenges in exposure monitoring. Because most types of PPE work by acting as a barrier to hazardous agents, healthcare personnel face challenges posed by barrier materials, including having difficulties in verbal communications and interactions with patients and family members, maintaining tactile sensitivity through gloves, and addressing physiological burdens.

Some types of PPE are used routinely by clinicians as part of standard infection control precautions designed to protect both the healthcare professional and the patient from disease acquisition. CDC has developed a tiered approach to infection control precautions that is detailed and reviewed by HICPAC. Standard precautions[5] (first tier) are applied to the care of all patients and include the use of gloves and hand hygiene. The second tier of precautions is used in cases where patients have documented or presumed infections or conditions that could be transmitted to healthcare personnel. The details of these transmission-based precautions are specific to situations with the potential for contact, airborne, or droplet transmission of infectious agents as defined by HICPAC (Siegel et al., 2007). Care of patients with suspected respiratory infections with viral agents—such as respiratory syncytial virus, adenovirus, parainfluenza, influenza, or human metapneumovirus—requires the use of contact and droplet precautions to protect the healthcare worker from exposure to droplet spray and contact. The guideline further notes that once adenovirus and influenza have been ruled out, droplet precautions can be discontinued (Siegel et al., 2007, p. 121).

As noted in the 2008 report, opportunities abound to provide innovative approaches that could improve PPE design to better fit healthcare needs, incorporate an emphasis on worker safety, and integrate worker and patient safety efforts. In discussing the issues relevant to the use of PPE by healthcare personnel, the committee identified a set of criteria as a starting point for decisions on selecting and using PPE. PPE for healthcare personnel should

- effectively reduce risks of disease or injury to healthcare personnel;

---

[5]See Siegel et al. (2007) for details on PPE used at each level of precautions.

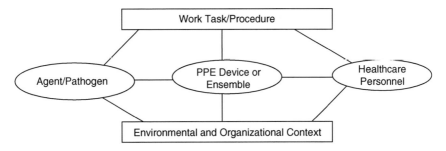

FIGURE 1-1 The major components and factors involved in the use of personal protective equipment in health care.

- minimize negative interactions with or effects on patients and their families and caregivers;
- be acceptable and usable by healthcare personnel in their day-to-day tasks, including ease of communication and comfort;
- be practical regarding issues of cost, time, and training; and
- be appropriate to the occupational risk being encountered.

In developing the report, the committee considered the issues relevant to the pathogen (virus), the device, and the worker while realizing it needed to keep in mind the various work tasks of healthcare personnel, the safety culture, and other organizational issues regarding where and how they work, and the broader policy and regulatory issues. Figure 1-1 is a depiction of the major components or factors involved in PPE use in health care.

OVERVIEW OF INFLUENZA AND OTHER VIRAL RESPIRATORY DISEASES

This report draws on the 2009–2010 experience with H1N1 influenza A. However, a brief background section is included here to set the context for the report and to broaden the discussion to include other viral respiratory diseases. Although not the focus of this report, bacterial pathogens may also be transmitted via respiratory aerosols.

Influenza is a serious respiratory illness caused by infection with influenza type A or type B virus. Each year, more than 200,000 U.S.

hospitalizations result from seasonal influenza and its complications (Thompson et al., 2004). Estimates of the number of deaths in the United States associated annually with seasonal influenza (from 1976 to 2007) ranged from a low of about 3,300 to a high of about 49,000, with most of the excess mortality in persons 65 years and older (Thompson et al., 2010). Cases of influenza peak during the winter months in each hemisphere. The influenza A virus is categorized by the subtypes of its major surface glycoproteins: hemagglutinin and neuraminidase.[6] The influenza virus undergoes frequent changes in antigenicity. Vaccines and antiviral medications have been developed to prevent or mitigate the disease, although major challenges remain, particularly in determining the appropriate viral strain to be included in the annual vaccine.

In contrast to seasonal occurrences of influenza, global outbreaks or pandemics occur more rarely. In the twentieth century, influenza pandemics occurred in 1918, 1957, and 1968. The highest mortality was in the 1918 pandemic, which is estimated to have resulted in 675,000 deaths in the United States and 50 million or more deaths worldwide (Johnson and Mueller, 2002; Morens and Fauci, 2007). The 2009 H1N1 virus was first detected in Mexico in April 2009 and quickly appeared in the United States. Although the incidence was high and difficult to measure (as only a small percentage are laboratory-confirmed cases), it was milder than expected and more likely to affect people under age 65 than seasonal influenza (CDC, 2010e). In the United States, CDC estimates there were between 43 and 89 million cases of H1N1 between April 2009 and April 10, 2010, with an estimate of 8,870 to 18,300 deaths related to the 2009 H1N1 (CDC, 2010e).

In late April 2009, CDC began to release 25 percent of the supplies in the Strategic National Stockpile that could be needed to protect against the influenza virus and treat influenza patients. This equated to approximately 11 million regimens of antiviral drugs and 39 million pieces of PPE, including face masks, respirators, gowns, gloves, and face shields (allocations were based on each state's population) (CDC, 2010a).

Other viral respiratory diseases are also a concern for the health and safety of healthcare personnel, ranging from emerging diseases, such as severe acute respiratory syndrome (SARS), to the highly prevalent and seasonal respiratory syncytial virus (RSV). In 2003, worldwide attention focused on an outbreak of infections caused by a previously unrecognized coronavirus that resulted in SARS. Healthcare personnel, partic-

---

[6]Hemagglutinin mediates the binding of influenza virus to the cells. Neuraminidase is involved in the release of virus from infected cells.

ularly those not using PPE and other infection control practices, were among the vulnerable groups (CDC, 2003). RSV infections are especially a concern in infants and older adults. The symptoms of RSV infections are similar to other respiratory diseases, including influenza, and transmission routes of RSV include direct and indirect contact, droplet spray, and aerosol routes. Each year in the United States, 75,000 to 125,000 infants are hospitalized with RSV (CDC, 2010d), and their care may involve many types of healthcare personnel.

Having recently been through the 2009–2010 experience with H1N1 influenza, the committee is well aware of the ongoing challenges and controversies surrounding PPE for healthcare personnel. Lessons continue to be learned regarding strategies to address why some healthcare personnel do not use preventive measures that are available and effective, particularly because preventing disease has implications for both improving the health of the workers and their patients. At this time, it is particularly important to build on the recent H1N1 experience and take the actions needed to address the research and policy questions that will allow the healthcare community to be better prepared for the next epidemic or pandemic. While the optimist can seek comfort in the fact that progress has been made in the past several years, the pragmatist must wonder about the rate of progress (or lack thereof) on such a critical issue that potentially threatens the security and economic well-being of the nation and the world. Experience has shown that relevant research on these issues wanes between pandemics. Avoiding that scenario this time is crucial to resolving the research questions and setting evidence-based policies in place.

DEFINING AN INTEGRATED APPROACH
TO PPE RESEARCH

Providing care to ill or injured patients involves a range of potentially hazardous exposures for healthcare personnel. Current infection control precautions address this challenge by providing guidance on PPE and other precautions that varies depending on the mode of transmission of the pathogen. The ultimate goal would be to have definitive information that would match the appropriate type of PPE with the pathogen, its mode of transmission, the infectious dose, and its risk to healthcare personnel. In many cases in industrial settings, this level of specificity is available for chemical exposures, although other industrial settings with unknown or mixed exposures continue to pose challenges. Reaching that point for protecting healthcare personnel will require concerted research efforts.

This report explores an integrated approach that addresses the full spectrum of research (from basic research to policy research) and translates research findings into improvements in the standards of healthcare practice (Figure 1-2). This approach ensures that basic science initiatives are fully explored, while also addressing clinical needs and testing the results in real-world settings, with the expectation that adaptations will be made and tested along the way. Feedback loops to prior stages are also critically important. Such an integrated approach calls for active collaboration and discourse among scientists and clinicians who may not have had previous interactions.

Chapters 2 to 5 each begin with a short summary of the relevant discussion of the 2008 report, followed by an update of recent research efforts outlining the state of progress in that area, and concluding with the committee's recommendations on research needs and directions. The committee examined four major areas of research:

- transmission of influenza and other viral respiratory diseases and the use of PPE in preventing transmission (Chapter 2);

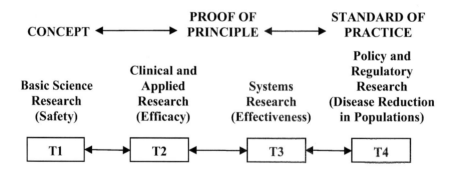

FIGURE 1-2 An integrated system moving research into practice, depicting the translation of research from basic science research (T1) through policy and regulatory research (T4).
SOURCE: Adapted from Henderson and Palmore (2010) with permission from University of Chicago Press.

- design and engineering of PPE to be effective and wearable (Chapter 3);
- use of PPE by healthcare personnel (Chapter 4); and
- policy, standards setting, and certification (Chapter 5).

The report covers PPE issues that are relevant to preventing the transmission of a number of viral respiratory diseases; however, much of the recent research and discussion is focused on influenza and, as a result, influenza is the primary disease discussed in the report. The priorities noted throughout this report are to determine the type of PPE needed for given exposures and to move effective, wearable, and innovative PPE products through the basic research and initial testing phases and on to active use and evaluation by the worker community.

REFERENCES

BLS (Bureau of Labor Statistics). 2010. *Career guide to industries, 2010-2011 edition: Healthcare.* http://www.bls.gov/oco/cg/cgs035.htm (accessed November 19, 2010).

CDC (Centers for Disease Control and Prevention). 2003. Cluster of severe acute respiratory syndrome cases among protected health-care workers—Toronto, Canada, April 2003. *Morbidity and Mortality Weekly Report* 52(19):433-436.

———. 2010a. *The 2009 H1N1 pandemic: Summary highlights, April 2009-April 2010.* http://cdc.gov/h1n1flu/cdcresponse.htm (accessed November 19, 2010).

———. 2010b. *2010-11 influenza prevention and control recommendations: Additional information about vaccination of specific populations.* http://www.cdc.gov/flu/professionals/acip/specificpopulations.htm (accessed November 30, 2010).

———. 2010c. *Prevention strategies for seasonal influenza in healthcare settings.* http://www.cdc.gov/flu/professionals/infectioncontrol/healthcare settings.htm (accessed December 20, 2010).

———. 2010d. Respiratory syncytial virus activity—United States, July 2008-December 2009. *Morbidity and Mortality Weekly Report* 59(8):230-233.

———. 2010e. *Updated CDC estimates of 2009 H1N1 influenza cases, hospitalizations and deaths in the United States, April 2009-April 10, 2010.* http://www.cdc.gov/h1n1flu/estimates_2009_h1n1.htm (accessed November 19, 2010).

Fiore, A. E., C. B. Bridges, and N. J. Cox. 2009. Seasonal influenza vaccines. *Current Topics in Microbiology and Immunology* 333:43-82.

Henderson, D. K., and T. N. Palmore. 2010. Critical gaps in knowledge of the epidemiology and pathophysiology of healthcare-associated infections. *Infection Control and Hospital Epidemiology* 31(Suppl. 1):S4-S6.

IOM (Institute of Medicine). 2008. *Preparing for an influenza pandemic: Personal protective equipment for healthcare workers.* Washington, DC: The National Academies Press.

———. 2009. *Respiratory protection for healthcare workers in the workplace against novel H1N1 Influenza A: A letter report.* Washington, DC: The National Academies Press.

Johnson, N. P., and J. Mueller. 2002. Updating the accounts: Global mortality of the 1918-1920 "Spanish" influenza pandemic. *Bulletin of the History of Medicine* 76(1):105-115.

Morens, D. M., and A. S. Fauci. 2007. The 1918 influenza pandemic: Insights for the 21st century. *Journal of Infectious Diseases* 195(7):1018-1028.

NIOSH (National Institute for Occupational Safety and Health). 2007. *Evidence for the National Academies' review of the NIOSH personal protective technology program.* http://www.cdc.gov/niosh/nas/ppt/pdfs/PPT_EvPkg_090707_FinalR.pdf (accessed November 30, 2010).

OSHA (Occupational Safety and Health Administration). 2002. *OSHA fact sheet: Personal protective equipment.* http://www.osha.gov/OshDoc/data_General_Facts/ppe-factsheet.pdf (accessed November 30, 2010).

Siegel, J. D., E. Rhinehart, M. Jackson, L. Chiarello, and the Healthcare Infection Control Practices Advisory Committee. 2007. *2007 guideline for isolation precautions: Preventing transmission of infectious agents in healthcare settings.* http://www.cdc.gov/hicpac/pdf/isolation/Isolation2007.pdf (accessed December 20, 2010).

Thompson, M., D. Shay, H. Zhou, C. Bridges, P. Cheng, E. Burns, J. Bresee, and N. Cox. 2010. Estimates of deaths associated with seasonal influenza—United States, 1976–2007. *Morbidity and Mortality Weekly Report* 59(33):1057-1062.

Thompson, W. W., D. K. Shay, E. Weintraub, L. Brammer, C. B. Bridges, N. J. Cox, and K. Fukuda. 2004. Influenza-associated hospitalizations in the United States. *Journal of the American Medical Association* 292(11):1333-1340.

Treanor, J. J., K. Kotloff, R. F. Betts, R. Belshe, F. Newman, D. Iacuzio, J. Wittes, and M. Bryant. 1999. Evaluation of trivalent, live, cold-adapted (CAIV-T) and inactivated (TIV) influenza vaccines in prevention of virus infection and illness following challenge of adults with wild-type influenza A (H1N1), A (H3N2), and B viruses. *Vaccine* 18(9-10):899-906.

2

Understanding the Risk
to Healthcare Personnel

Interest in the transmission of influenza viruses has increased in recent years due to the ongoing zoonotic infection of humans with avian
H5N1 influenza viruses and the pandemic spread of a swine-like H1N1
strain in 2009. In particular, the recognition that person-to-person transmission is a major criterion that must be met for *pandemic* infection has
stimulated research into the mechanisms by which influenza viruses are
transmitted and what factors enhance or interfere with this transmission.
In considering preventive efforts to avoid viral respiratory disease transmission, the committee emphasizes the importance of the use of a range
of hazard controls, including vaccination, to protect healthcare personnel.

This chapter provides a synopsis of the discussion in the 2008 report
regarding influenza transmission followed by an overview of recent
(2007 to mid-2010) research on viral respiratory disease transmission.
Studies on personal protective equipment (PPE) use to prevent viral respiratory disease transmission are also reviewed. The chapter concludes
with the committee's thoughts on immediate research needs and long-
term research opportunities.

BACKGROUND AND CONTEXT
FROM THE 2008 REPORT

The prior Institute of Medicine report examined research studies conducted through 2007 on the modes of influenza transmission and highlighted the paucity of data on the relative contributions of each to the risk
of illness in the community or clinical setting. A major challenge in research on this issue has been the lack of consistency in the use of terms

to describe particle size and to describe potential transmission routes (Box 2-1). As research efforts move forward, agreement is needed on terminology to be used so that studies can be compared. Box 2-1 provides the definitions used by the committee throughout the report, including in describing earlier studies. The terms and definitions of the transmission routes were developed at a recent Centers for Disease Control and Prevention (CDC) workshop (David Weissman, personal communication, CDC, November 2010) and are provided as a starting point. These are operational

---

BOX 2-1
Terminology—Particle Size and Transmission Routes

As noted above, the terms and definitions here are used to frame the discussion, and efforts are needed to reach consensus agreement among the many relevant areas of research and clinical care.

Particle Size:
- *Respirable particles*–particles with $d_a \leq 10$ μm that can be inhaled and penetrate to the alveolar region; although a substantial fraction deposit in the alveolar region, they deposit throughout the respiratory tract. These are the equivalent of "droplet nuclei."
- *Inspirable particles*–particles with 10 μm $\leq d_a \leq 100$ μm, which can be inhaled but cannot penetrate to the alveolar region; nearly all deposit in the head airways region.

Transmission Routes:
- *Contact transmission:*
  - *Direct contact transmission* occurs when the virus is transferred by contact from an infected person to another person without a contaminated intermediate object.
  - *Indirect contact transmission* involves the transfer of viral agents by contact with a contaminated intermediate object.
- *Droplet spray transmission:* Person-to-person transmission of the virus through the air by droplet sprays. A key feature is deposition by impaction on exposed mucous membranes.
- *Aerosol transmission:* Person-to-person transmission of influenza or other respiratory viruses through the air by aerosols in the inspirable (inhalable) size range or smaller. Particles are small enough to be inhaled into the oronasopharynx and distally into the trachea and lung.

NOTE: d_a = aerodynamic diameter. Terminology regarding particles with $d_a > 100$ μm is needed.
SOURCES: Nicas and Jones (2009); Personal communication, D. Weissman, November 2010.

definitions and are not CDC policy. The definitions of particle size are adapted from a set of definitions described by Nicas and Jones (2009). Further work is needed on standardization of terminology. A common set of definitions accepted by the industrial hygiene, infectious disease, and healthcare communities would be most helpful in discussing future research and policy.

Much of the discussion regarding influenza transmission has focused on the continuum between droplet spray and aerosol transmission, as well as on the role of contact transmission and the potential for transmission through inoculation of the conjunctivae. Aerosol transmission, an issue in healthcare settings where patients have diseases such as tuberculosis and measles, can occur at a short range between persons but can also involve infectious agents carried for longer distances by air currents. Fabian and colleagues (2008) collected exhaled breath of patients with active influenza. In 4 of 12 subjects, exhaled breath contained influenza, and more than 87 percent of exhaled particles were < 1 μm.

One of the main reasons why there is no clear understanding of long-range transmission is because aerosol transmission of influenza and other respiratory viruses is difficult to study in human populations. To study long-range aerosol transmission properly, the background prevalence of the disease would need to be low in the community, and many other factors would need to be controlled to rule out other transmission routes, such as droplet spray and contact (Tellier, 2009). Production of aerosols also varies by individual; some individuals produce large amounts of bioaerosols in coughs, sneezes, and even tidal breathing, while others do not. Therefore, some individuals may be more or less likely to transmit influenza infection or other viral respiratory diseases via aerosols.

Context is likely to play an important role in shaping the importance of these transmission pathways in relation to illness occurrence. Researchers have shown that contextual factors may include environment, humidity, temperature, number and types of fomites, air flow, age of susceptible and infected populations, and number of individuals and their interactions within space. Biological factors that may influence transmission include virus strain characteristics, human physiology, immune status, and genetic susceptibility of the host.

Modifications to the living environment have the potential to reduce the transmission of influenza virus or other respiratory viral agents. These modifications include increasing the rate of air exchange, using non-recirculated air, irradiating air prior to recirculation, and changing absolute humidity (Lowen et al., 2007; Shaman et al., 2010). Increased air exchange is expected to affect transmission by an aerosol route through a reduction in the concentration of infectious particles in the air. Because both temperature and humidity are known to impact the stability of influenza viruses in an aerosol (Harper, 1961, 1963; Hemmes et al., 1960; Schaffer et al., 1976), interventions to reduce transmission by altering these environmental conditions may be useful.

Influenza A transmission has been studied in various animal species—including mice, guinea pigs, monkeys, and ferrets—with variable results. These studies show that animals develop influenza infection, and most demonstrate the possible role of aerosol transmission. Experiments performed in the 1930s demonstrated that influenza virus–naïve, asymptomatic ferrets that were caged with influenza virus–infected ferrets would subsequently develop disease and that, even in the absence of experimental infection, ferrets occasionally displayed an influenza-like illness, after which they became immune to subsequent virus inoculation (Francis and Magill, 1935; Smith et al., 1933). Andrewes and Glover (1941) demonstrated transmission using an experimental design in which air flowed from infected to naïve ferrets through a tube containing S- and U-shaped bends, which would be expected to allow the transfer of only small (< 5 μm) respirable particles. In hamsters, by contrast, transmission of influenza viruses appeared to depend on contact between infected and exposed animals (Ali et al., 1982). A series of experiments with mice in the 1960s also provided some evidence suggesting aerosol transmission (Schulman, 1968; Schulman and Kilbourne, 1962). More recently, the guinea pig has been successfully used to study influenza transmission (Lowen et al., 2006).

Transmission among humans has been studied less. Early volunteer studies found that infection via inhalation of respirable particles requires considerably less virus than infection via droplets placed on the nasal membranes (Alford et al., 1966; Couch et al., 1971, 1974; Douglas, 1975). Several observational studies of naturally occurring influenza provided insights into the challenges of studying transmission modes. One of the most well-known incidents of an influenza A outbreak happened among passengers on a grounded airplane (Gregg, 1980; Moser et al., 1979). An observational study of 49 passengers delayed on a 737 jet for 3 hours and exposed to an index case with influenza suggested aerosol transmission. Within 72 hours, 72 percent of the passengers became ill. Specimens from 31 of the 38 cases were cultured and found to have similar isolates. A second airline travel–associated outbreak also suggested aerosol transmission with a 37 percent attack rate and wide seating distribution of secondary cases throughout the aircraft (Klontz et al., 1989). More recent studies of airline travel indicate close-proximity transmission (Baker et al., 2010; Han et al., 2009; Ooi et al., 2010), which could occur via one or more routes. Newer airplanes have more laminar air flow and improved filters over older planes, which may reduce long-range aerosol transmission. Studies examining how air flow may help prevent transmission of viral respiratory diseases in closed and crowded settings, such as an airplane, are warranted.

Wong and colleagues (2010) recently reported a nosocomial outbreak of seasonal influenza in an acute-ward setting that appeared to be attributed to aerosol transmission. An aerosol-generating device was used on the influenza index case patient. At the same time, the authors identified an imbalance in the indoor airflow that likely created a directional dispersion of air and potentially carried influenza aerosols to other areas of the ward. Other patients were infected following a temporal and spatial pattern of air flow originating from the index patient. Two of the staff also became ill even though they were required to adhere to strict hand hygiene and medical mask use.

Additional observational studies of human influenza have provided further descriptions of influenza outbreaks, but the findings do not clarify potential mechanisms of transmission (discussed in IOM, 2008). For example, Drinka and colleagues (1996, 2004) compared influenza rates in several buildings of a long-term care facility during several seasons of influenza. Their initial study found that persons working in buildings with ventilation systems that provided outside air had much lower infection rates than those working in buildings with partially recirculated air (Drinka et al., 1996). However, an update of this study found similar infection rates (Drinka et al., 2004). Reviews of other reported influenza outbreaks suggest droplet spray and contact transmission routes based on temporal and spatial patterns (Brankston et al., 2007; Cunney et al., 2000; Drinka et al., 1996; Morens and Rash, 1995).

Studies of the clinical effectiveness of PPE have had mixed results in preventing severe acute respiratory syndrome (SARS) or respiratory syncytial virus (RSV) infections (see Appendix C). Challenges in studies of this type include difficulties in retrospectively separating the effects of PPE from the effects of other infection control measures.

Specific issues regarding respiratory disease transmission to healthcare personnel have focused on medical procedures that have a potential for creating aerosols, and data are primarily available for SARS, not influenza. Fowler and colleagues (2004) observed a greater risk of developing SARS for physicians and nurses performing endotracheal intubation. Similarly, in a retrospective study of 43 nurses who worked in Toronto with SARS patients, Loeb and colleagues (2004) found that assisting during intubation, suctioning before intubation, and manipulating the oxygen mask were high-risk activities for acquiring SARS; wearing a face mask or N95 respirator was protective.

As stated throughout the 2008 report, establishing how influenza is transmitted and understanding the contribution of each mode of transmission is critical to preventing its spread and reducing morbidity and mortality due to influenza infection, especially in healthcare settings. The 2008 report outlined a number of questions that remained to be addressed regarding influenza transmission (IOM, 2008):

- *Questions regarding transmission mode, including:* What are the major modes of transmission? How much does each mode of transmission contribute individually or with other modes of transmission? What is the size distribution of particles expelled by infectious individuals, and how does that continuum of sizes affect transmission? Is the virus viable and infectious on fomites, and for how long? Are fomites a means of transmission, and are some more able to transmit than others?

- *Questions regarding infectivity, including:* Can infection take place through mucous membranes or conjunctiva exposure? What is the time sequence of infectivity?

- *Questions specific to transmission in healthcare settings, including:* What activities in the healthcare setting are associated with minimal or increased transmission? How distinct is transmission in different venues including health care, schools, and households?

- *Questions specific to the role of PPE in preventing or reducing transmission, including:* How effective is each type of PPE in reducing the risk of influenza transmission? How effective are face masks? What innovations regarding PPE are needed to enhance effectiveness? What is the impact on transmission risk when patients wear face masks?

- *Questions specific to other potential forms of prevention, including:* What is the role of ultraviolet (UV) light, humidity, temperature, pressure differentials, air flow and exchange, and ventilation in preventing transmission?

The 2008 report concluded its discussion regarding research on influenza transmission with a recommendation that a Global Influenza Research Network should be initiated and supported. This network would facilitate an understanding of the transmission and prevention of seasonal and pandemic influenza, with priority funding given to short-term clinical and laboratory studies. Furthermore, the recommendation stressed the need to develop rigorous, evidence-based research protocols and implementation plans for clinical studies for use during an influenza pandemic (IOM, 2008).

UPDATE ON RECENT RESEARCH

In the 3 years since the writing of the prior report (IOM, 2008), research efforts continue to examine the various routes of transmission and explore approaches to preventing transmission. The following section provides an overview of recent research (2007 to mid-2010) and describes animal studies, environmental monitoring and persistence studies, transmission modeling studies, and human studies. The literature searches on disease transmission conducted by the committee focused on influenza. Searches of bibliographic databases for studies on PPE use and transmission were broader and incorporated other viral respiratory diseases; only a few recent studies on other viral respiratory diseases were identified, however, and those are discussed and referenced in this report.

Animal Studies

Animal models complement epidemiological approaches by allowing the examination of influenza virus transmission from an infected to a susceptible host under well-controlled conditions. The ferret and guinea pig models are the current models of choice in influenza studies. Ferrets are naturally susceptible to infection with human influenza viruses, and these viruses transmit among them, making the ferret the current gold-standard animal model for the study of influenza. Prompted by the need for a more convenient animal model than the ferret in which to study transmission, the guinea pig was recently developed as such a model host (Lowen et al., 2006). Although signs of disease are generally not observed in influenza virus–infected guinea pigs, these animals are highly susceptible to infection with human strains, and human influenza viruses transmit efficiently from one guinea pig to another.

Animal Models on Modes of Transmission

The relative contributions of the various modes by which influenza viruses transmit is currently a subject of debate in the field. In the context of experimental studies using animals, transmission by the contact route is normally modeled by placing infected and naïve animals into the same cage together. It is important to note, however, that this set-up does not allow one to distinguish transmission by a contact route from short-range spread mediated by an aerosol. To study transmission specifically by inspirable or respirable aerosols, animals are placed into separate cages so that air exchange can occur among them, but they cannot touch. Although this arrangement rules out contact-based transmission, when cages are placed in close proximity (as is usually the case), transmission may proceed via the droplet spray or aerosol modes.

Transmission of human seasonal and 2009 H1N1 pandemic strains among either ferrets or guinea pigs occurs efficiently using both experimental designs, indicating that transmission among ferrets and guinea pigs can proceed in the absence of direct or indirect contact among animals (recent studies include Lowen et al., 2006, 2007, 2008; Maines et al., 2009; Munster et al., 2009; Steel et al., 2010; Tumpey et al., 2007). In addition, evidence for transmission of influenza viruses by the aerosol route has been obtained in the ferret and guinea pig models; early work in ferrets (Andrewes and Glover, 1941) and recent experiments performed in guinea pigs (Mubareka et al., 2009) demonstrate transmission over a distance of up to 3.5 feet.

Recent attempts to model influenza virus transmission in BALB/c mice have been unsuccessful (Lowen et al., 2006); nevertheless, a mouse model was used by Schulman and Kilbourne to study transmission in the 1960s (Schulman, 1968; Schulman and Kilbourne, 1962). Because of the inefficiency of transmission and the low susceptibility of mice to human influenza viruses that have not been serially adapted in this host, currently the mouse model is not used widely for research on influenza virus transmission. Hamsters are also not in widespread use as a model for influenza virus infection, but Ali and colleagues (1982) showed that certain human influenza isolates transmitted well when infected and naïve hamsters were housed in the same cage; transmission in the absence of contact was not, however, observed.

The potential for contact with contaminated surfaces to mediate influenza virus transmission among guinea pigs was examined by Mubareka and colleagues (2009). Naïve guinea pigs were placed in cages that either had previously housed an acutely infected animal or had been contaminated with high titers of influenza virus through direct application onto non-porous cage surfaces. In the former case, approximately 20 percent of exposed animals contracted infection, while with the latter design, no exposed animals became infected (Mubareka et al., 2009). When these results are compared to the high efficiency of transmission of the same virus by the aerosol route, they suggest that—at least in the guinea pig model—spread via fomites makes a minor contribution to the overall transmission of influenza viruses.

Relationships Between Transmission and Symptoms, Timing Post-Infection, and Shedding Titers

Because of their potential to produce infectious aerosols, coughing and sneezing are generally thought to promote transmission (Tumpey et al., 2007). Evidence against a critical role for sneezing and coughing arises from the guinea pig model: Although these animals do not sneeze or cough following influenza virus infection, viral spread is efficient among guinea pigs (Lowen et al., 2007). Influenza viruses have been isolated from the air surrounding infected guinea pigs (Mubareka et al., 2009) and even mice (Schulman, 1967); this virus is most likely expelled into the environment through normal breathing (Fabian et al., 2008).

The timing of transmission events relative to initial infection of donor animals has not been examined closely (through the use of defined exposure periods) in the ferret or guinea pig models; the serial collection of nasal wash samples over the course of exposure does, however, allow an estimate of the time of transmission to be made. In the guinea pig model after exposure by contact and aerosol routes, virus was detected initially in the nasal washings of exposed animals at 1–3 days and 3–5 days, respectively (Lowen et al., 2006, 2007, 2008, 2009; Steel et al., 2009). The infection of exposed ferrets occurs with similar timing by contact and aerosol routes: Initial detection of virus in the nasal passages of exposed animals usually occurs between 1 and 3 days post-exposure (Itoh et al., 2009; Maines et al., 2006, 2009; Tumpey et al., 2007). Variations in transmissibility among differing strains of influenza viruses do not show a strong correlation with differences in peak shedding titers (Maines et al., 2006, 2009; Mubareka et al., 2009; Steel et al., 2009; Tumpey et al., 2007), suggesting that, although efficient growth in the upper respiratory tract is most likely required for an influenza virus to transmit, additional criteria must be met for transmission to proceed.

Relative Transmissibility of Influenza Viruses Derived from Different Host Species

Viral strain and subtype specific differences in influenza virus transmission have been observed in recent studies of animal models. One strength of both the ferret and guinea pig models is that influenza viruses adapted to human hosts generally transmit more efficiently than avian-, swine-, or mouse-adapted strains. Thus, the low pathogenic avian strains A/duck/Alberta/35/1976 (H1N1) and A/duck/Ukraine/1963 (H3N8) did not transmit among guinea pigs, while certain highly pathogenic H5N1 influenza viruses have been observed to transmit among co-caged guinea pigs to a limited extent (Gao et al., 2009; Steel et al., 2009). Swine influenza isolates of the H3 subtypes transmitted with 25 percent efficiency by the aerosol route among guinea pigs (Steel et al., 2010). By contrast, human H3N2 subtype viruses, as well as the H1N1 pandemic strain, generally transmit to all exposed guinea pigs by either contact or aerosol routes (Lowen et al., 2006; Steel et al., 2010). Overall, seasonal H1N1 subtype viruses have been found to transmit less efficiently among guinea pigs than epidemic strains of the H3N2 subtype (Mubareka et al., 2009). A similar pattern of transmissibility is observed in the ferret model: Avian influenza viruses do not transmit to exposed animals by an aerosol route (Tumpey et al., 2007; Van Hoeven et al., 2009), but some low and highly pathogenic strains do transmit by contact to a limited extent (Belser et al., 2008; Maines et al., 2006; Sorrell et al., 2009; Van Hoeven et al., 2009; Wan et al., 2008). Human seasonal strains of both H3N2 and H1N1 subtypes transmit readily among ferrets (Itoh et al., 2009; Maines et al., 2006, 2009; Wan et al., 2008), and the pandemic H1N1 strain has been observed to transmit with similar efficiency (Itoh et al., 2009; Munster et al., 2009) or somewhat lower efficiency (Maines et al., 2009) by an aerosol route than seasonal influenza viruses.

Interventions: Blocking Influenza Virus Transmission in Animal Models

Interventions that offer the potential to limit transmission of influenza viruses in healthcare settings include vaccination; the prophylactic and therapeutic use of antiviral drugs; non-pharmaceutical interventions, such as the use of good hand hygiene and PPE; use of source control; cohorting the patients; and modifications to the indoor environment. Changes in transmission achieved through vaccination were studied in the guinea pig model, and it was found that transmission could be abrogated through vaccination. This was the case whether the vaccinated animals were the donors or recipients in the transmission experiment. Vaccination was particularly effective in blocking spread if sterilizing immunity was achieved (as was seen using a live attenuated vaccine), but transmission was also reduced following suboptimal vaccination[1] (Lowen et al., 2009). Also in guinea pigs, twice-daily treatment with oseltamivir reduced titers shed from the upper respiratory tract of treated donor guinea pigs and, in turn, prevented transmission to untreated aerosol contacts. This is similar to recent and past studies of prophylactic treatment of household contacts of infected persons that has been found to be very effective (Halloran et al., 2007; Hayden et al., 2000, 2004; Monto et al., 2002; Welliver et al., 2001).

Research in the past several years has demonstrated in the guinea pig model that transmission between animals in separate cages occurs with lower frequency (or not at all) when the surrounding air is warm (30°C) or maintained at high (80 percent) or intermediate (50 percent) relative humidities (Lowen et al., 2007, 2008). Although field studies are required to translate these findings to the human situation, they suggest that the modification of relative humidity in healthcare settings may be a means of controlling the spread of influenza virus infection. The impact of UV treatment of air on influenza viral spread has not been assessed in an animal model; if transmission proceeds at least in part by an aerosol route, however, such treatment is expected to be effective.

---

[1]The authors describe suboptimal vaccines as those that may provide only partial protection against the disease but are effective at limiting transmission (Lowen et al., 2009).

Environmental Monitoring and Persistence Studies

Air Monitoring

To learn more about the distribution of aerosol influenza virus in an urgent care setting, two studies have recently been conducted. A study by Blachere and colleagues (2009) of real-time polymerase chain reaction (RT-PCR) identified the presence of aerosolized influenza in several areas of an emergency department, including a waiting room, a reception area, and personal samplers placed on physicians. On 3 of 6 separate days, aerosolized influenza A virus was detected. Half of the influenza particles were found to be in the respirable size range. The follow-up study by Lindsley and colleagues (2010a) looked at both influenza and RSV. Seventeen percent of the stationary samplers contained influenza A ribonucleic acid (RNA), and 32 percent contained RSV. Nineteen percent and 38 percent of clinical staff samplers contained influenza A and RSV RNA, respectively. A correlation was found between samplers that contained influenza and presence of patients who were positive for influenza (r = 0.77). A slightly smaller proportion of the influenza A RNA was in particles ≤ 4.1 μm in aerodynamic diameter (42 percent) compared with the earlier study by Blachere and colleagues (2009) (53 percent). These studies indicate that aerosolized particles exist in this specific urgent care setting. However, the viability of the influenza viruses was not ascertained, and therefore it is not possible to quantify the importance of the identified aerosol particles to transmission in the hospital setting.

A recent study by Lindsley and colleagues (2010b) showed that 84 percent (32/38) of influenza-positive patients had influenza viral RNA in their cough aerosols as identified by a National Institute for Occupational Safety and Health two-stage bioaerosol cyclone sampler or an SKC Bio-Sampler. Of the influenza viral RNA detected, 65 percent was contained in particles in the respirable range (< 4 μm), suggesting that these particles could be inhaled and deposited in the alveolar region of the lungs. Viable virus was detected in the cough aerosols of some infected patients. A limitation of the collection system was the inability to collect larger particles. Therefore, this study was unable to quantify the proportion of small versus large particles or the total amount of viral material contained in the cough of an influenza-infected patient.

Fomite Persistence

Studies examining fomite contamination have focused largely on virus survivability on environmental surfaces. The type of fomite surface appears to play a significant role in influenza virus survival with low survival times on porous materials, such as paper and cloth, ranging from 8 to 12 hours and on non-porous materials, such as stainless steel and plastic, ranging from 24 to 72 hours (Boone and Gerba, 2007). Other factors likely to affect survival of influenza on fomites include cleanliness and moisture. In experimental studies reviewed by Boone and Gerba, transfer of influenza virus to the hands occurred up to 24 hours after contaminating stainless steel fomites with influenza virus. Hands appear not to be a very hospitable environment for influenza, with viral decay occurring within the first 5 minutes of fomite-to-hand transfer. Nonetheless, if hands are continually inoculated by a touch to contaminated fomites, direct infection is likely. In the case of commonly touched fomites, influenza virus may be transferred from the fomite to the hands of a human host through consistent contact. As noted in an earlier study, among clinicians, 1 in 3 healthcare professionals rubbed their eyes and 42 percent picked their nose per 1-hour observation, suggesting that self-inoculation of influenza virus among these healthcare personnel would be likely if hands became contaminated in the hospital environment (Boone and Gerba, 2007; Hendley et al., 1973).

The significance of fomites in the spread of respiratory disease has been assessed through experimental seeding studies and assessments of inactivation rates (Boone and Gerba, 2007). Of the inactivation rates reviewed across a range of respiratory viruses (rhinovirus, RSV, coronaviruses, parainfluenza virus, avian influenza, and influenza A and B viruses), avian influenza and influenza A viruses had the lowest $\log_{10}$ reductions per hour. The $\log_{10}$ reduction per hour on non-porous fomites were 22 and 45 times lower for avian influenza and influenza A virus, respectively, compared to RSV, which had the highest $\log_{10}$ reduction per hour on surfaces. The only other respiratory virus with similar survivability as influenza on non-porous surfaces was rhinovirus, which can also survive for more than 24 hours. Avian influenza virus, in particular, was shown to have high survival rates on both porous and non-porous surfaces, including stainless steel, latex gloves, and cotton—as long as 144 hours. Survival on fomites, therefore, is much longer than what has been observed for human influenza survival in artificially produced aerosols, where rates ranged from 6 to 16 hours (Brankston et al., 2007; Mitchell and Guerin, 1972; Mitchell et al., 1968).

In a recent experimental study, coronavirus was detected on PPE at a minimum of 4 hours following initial exposure (Casanova et al., 2010). N95 respirators, contact isolation gowns, and latex gloves all had detectable virus 24 hours after exposure. The authors concluded that coronaviruses were able to survive on hospital PPE longer than the duration of contact with an infected patient. Far fewer observational studies have been done on influenza and other respiratory viruses on surfaces and PPE in the clinical setting. There are some developments in antimicrobial masks, but the utility and risks associated with these embedded materials are unclear. For example, Li and colleagues (2006) examined the antimicrobial activity of nanoparticle material with a mixture of silver nitrate and titanium dioxide for reducing bacteria on N95 respirators. There were large reductions in *S. aureus* and *E. coli* after 48 hours of incubation, but whether this material would have any activity against influenza was unclear because no respiratory viruses were tested in the study (Li et al., 2006). Macias and colleagues (2009) examined the extent of 2009 H1N1 contamination on the hands of healthcare personnel and patients and on environmental surfaces in a hospital in Mexico. The computer mouse, hands, and bed rails were all found to be positive for the influenza virus, but viability of the virus was not assessed. Studies have also examined the role of the contact transmission route in the transfer of rhinovirus and RSV (Gwaltney et al., 1978; Hall et al., 1980, 1981). Taken together, these experimental and observational studies support a role for the contaminated environment and PPE as a potential source of viable respiratory viruses, such as influenza. Nonetheless, no recent studies identified by the committee have examined whether infection can be transmitted directly from contact with a contaminated fomite.

Inactivation of Influenza A Viruses

A review by Weber and Stilianakis (2008) examined studies on the inactivation of influenza A viruses in the environment and the impact on modes of transmission. Currently little is known about inactivation of influenza virus. Experimental studies indicate that low relative humidity in heated indoor areas promotes influenza survival in the closed environment. However, the converse relationship has been observed outside of the United States, where outbreaks have occurred in tropical regions during hot and rainy months. Relative humidity does not independently predict virus survivability. Because of the variability in global outbreak patterns by relative humidity, some have argued that contact transmission may predominate in tropical climates whereas aerosol transmission is more common in temperate climates (Lowen and Palese, 2009). Modeling studies support a role of humidity in predicting disease outbreaks. Shaman and colleagues (2010) report that absolute humidity provided a robust correlate for seasonal variation in temperate climates.

Transmission Models

Although empirical studies have shown that influenza transmission is feasible by aerosol, droplet spray, and contact routes, the results of these studies have not provided a comprehensive understanding of the relative contribution of each mode in causing outbreaks. Mathematical models can be used as a method for testing hypotheses about the spread of respiratory infections (Brauer, 2009). Not all components of disease spread are measured in these models, but important parameters can be identified and estimated. Unfortunately, the lack of basic scientific data on transmission and survivability of influenza makes it very difficult to accurately determine the parameters for these models or to assess the fit of these models with available data. Many transmission models looking at the spread of influenza and other respiratory diseases include simulations that provide varying estimates on different modes of transmission, including the case reproductive number (R_0), social patterning, susceptibility, and influenza strain characteristics. The following summary of recent research in this area focuses on the key findings and assumptions inherent in these models in a way that may apply to healthcare personnel.

Multiple modes of influenza transmission have been explored using modeling information. Potential sources of influenza transmission to healthcare personnel through community and nosocomial exposures have also been modeled.

Models of the Dynamics of Influenza Transmission

Nicas and Jones (2009) examined the contribution of four modes of influenza transmission: hand contact; respirable particles (cough particles < 10 μm in diameter); inspirable particles (cough particles 10–100 μm in diameter); and droplet spray (> 100 μm in diameter). This study used two very different assumptions regarding infectivity: (1) the ratio of infectivity was 3,200:1 for influenza virus deposited in the lower respiratory tract compared to the upper respiratory tract, and (2) the ratio of infectivity was 1:1 for influenza virus deposited in the lower respiratory tract versus the upper respiratory tract. The infectivity ratio assumptions played a major role in determining which method of transmission was most likely to cause disease. Assuming a 3,200:1 infectivity ratio for influenza virus deposited in the lower respiratory tract compared with the upper respiratory tract, droplet spray accounted for 58 percent of the infection risk at low salivary viral concentrations, compared to 27 percent of the risk for fomite or hand contact and 14 percent of risk from respirable particles. Little is known about virus saliva concentrations in humans, which may vary widely.

As the salivary viral concentration increased, the risk of infection from droplet spray decreased, while the importance of hand contact in spreading disease increased. However, with a 1:1 ratio of infectivity in the lower versus upper respiratory tract, hand contact was the major driver of infection across all viral salivary concentrations (Nicas and Jones, 2009). The main measures assessed for reducing the risk of influenza transmission in the healthcare setting included hand washing, disposable gloves, and face masks to reduce touching the face. Measures for preventing infection caused by droplet spray included fluid-resistant masks and eye goggles or face shields. Besides social distancing, the model found that the most effective way to reduce respirable and inspirable particles included the use of an N95 filtering respirator and/or increasing the room ventilation. When the model used an infectivity ratio of 1:1, the research found that if influenza-positive individuals have a low concentration of salivary virus, healthcare personnel can significantly decrease the risk of transmission through simple methods, such as hand washing, standard surgical face masks with goggles, or face shields. At an infectivity ratio of 3,200:1, respirable particles would make up a substantial part of the risks, and respirators would be required.

Chen and colleagues (2009a) specifically assessed the dynamics of aerosol influenza transmission and found the volume of particles released from a sneeze were approximately three-fold higher than for a cough. Using an equation to estimate the total volume of particles had the following results: with cough, the highest volume occurred with a particle sized 5.8 μm (which would be classified as respirable particles by Nicas and Jones [2009]), leading to a volume of virus of 500×10^{-10} mL, and

26 μm for sneeze (classified as inspirable particles by Nicas and Jones), with a volume of virus of 3×10^{-7} mL. The predicted tissue culture infective dose$_{50}$ (TCID$_{50}$) for influenza was estimated to be 0.57 at 5.5 μm per cough 2.6 days after infection, and 264 per sneeze at 10 μm after 2.6 days. This model suggests that the TCID$_{50}$ produced by a sneeze is higher than that emanating from a cough.

A model of the risk of aerosol transmission was examined in the setting of a commuter train. Assuming the inhalation of aerosol infectious agents during a commute, the estimated R_0 was found to be 2.22 (geometric standard deviation [SD] = 1.53), with a specified number of air ventilation cycles per hour (Furuya, 2007). An exposure time of less than 30 minutes was found to reduce the likelihood of transmission, as were surgical masks to reduce droplet spray transmission (assuming a reduction in the risk of contaminated air inhaled by 40 percent), and high-efficiency particulate air masks (assuming a reduction in contaminated air inhaled by 97 percent) to reduce smaller particulate transmission. Of significance for healthcare personnel, doubling the number of air ventilation cycles per hour was found to reduce the risk of infection to $R_0 = 1$. Although not all healthcare settings are comparable to the close and extended proximity found on a commuter train, the effectiveness of increasing the number of air ventilation cycles per hour may be useful for reducing the likelihood of inhalation exposure to aerosol particles in the clinical setting. Other factors to consider in addition to ventilation would be the number of windows, number of stops, opening and closing of doors, and movement of people.

Models of Household Transmission

Household transmission models may be useful as a proxy for transmission within the healthcare setting. A single household model with two bedrooms and a common living quarter was used to assess the likelihood of influenza infection (Atkinson and Wein, 2008). The model included one infected individual, one primary caregiver, and two other household residents. The authors assumed that the death rate (rate of viral inactivation) on porous surfaces was more than one magnitude higher than the death rate on non-porous surfaces (0.12 per hour versus 1.78 per hour). The death rate of virus in the air was estimated to be 0.36 per hour. The authors assumed viral transmission occurred from the infected individual to the caregiver only within the infected individual's room, through un-

protected aerosol transmission with no deposition on surrounding surfaces. Transmission was assumed through close contact at the time of the
infected individual's emission, and that aerosol virus would be deposited
on either porous or non-porous surfaces. The authors then compared total
influenza virus shed, infectious dose likely to infect half of the population, and death rate of the viruses on different surfaces between influenza
virus and the rhinovirus. They found a higher total shed virus (1.93×10^5
$TCID_{50}$ compared to 1.57×10^5 $TCID_{50}$), higher $TCID_{50}$ required for respiratory epithelium (0.671 $TCID_{50}$ compared to 0.216 $TCID_{50}$), and much
higher $TCID_{50}$ for nose and eyes (500 $TCID_{50}$ compared to 0.032 $TCID_{50}$)
for influenza compared to rhinovirus. Although the death rate on hands
was much higher for the influenza virus (55.3 per hour) compared to rhinovirus (0.61 per hour), the death rate on porous and non-porous surfaces
was lower for influenza than rhinovirus. Atkinson and Wein (2008) concluded that aerosol transfer was the most likely mode of infection in the
described setting.

Models of Healthcare-Associated Infection

The committee was unable to identify any studies since 2007 that
modeled transmission of influenza within the hospital setting among
healthcare personnel. Earlier, Nicas and Sun (2006) modeled the risk of
transmissible respiratory diseases in a healthcare setting. The authors
provided an integrated method of examining transmission between infected individuals, contaminated environments, and direct patient-to-
healthcare worker exposure, which could be used as a template for an
influenza-specific model in the healthcare setting.

Models of Asymptomatic Carriers

The role of asymptomatic carriers in spreading influenza was examined using a Susceptible Exposed Infective Recovered model, with
two additional categories: asymptomatic and hospitalized (Hsu and
Hsieh, 2008). The model assumed that exposed individuals could either
become infectious, and then move toward a hospital or recover without
hospitalization, or become asymptomatic, and spread disease before recovering. Building on previous literature that up to a third of all influenza cases are asymptomatic, the authors assumed that asymptomatic

individuals contributed less to viral shedding as a result of a decrease in symptoms, such as coughing, that may spread disease. The authors found that the way that the public responds to information about an outbreak can reduce the number of influenza infections. However, due to asymptomatic influenza infections, community response alone cannot affect the basic dynamics of the model without additional steps, such as quarantine or other intervention measures, which were not included in the model because of additional complexities in their basic model. Therefore, with an asymptomatic subpopulation that is shedding virus, influenza can continue to persist within the community even with an R_0 of less than 1.

Human Challenge, Observational, and Clinical Studies

Infectivity, Viral Shedding, and Symptoms

The timing of infection and quantity of viral shedding obviously play a role in the spread of influenza. A meta-analysis of 56 volunteer challenge studies attempted to quantify the time of peak viral shedding among healthy human volunteers (Carrat et al., 2008b). Two different strains of virus were examined: influenza A/H1N1 strains (recovered earlier than 2009 H1N1) and influenza A/H3N2. In human volunteers, viral shedding showed a quick increase the first day following inoculation, with a maximum value reached after 2 days, and a return to baseline, on average, 8 days following inoculation. The first signs of shedding were observed in 83 percent of subjects 1 day after inoculation, 14 percent of subjects 2 days after inoculation, and 3 percent of subjects 3 days after inoculation, with an average duration of 1.1 days until viral shedding occurred. The mean duration of viral shedding was 4.80 days (95% confidence interval [CI] = 4.31, 5.29), with no significant difference in duration between H1N1 and H3N2 strains. One dose-varying study included in the meta-analysis found that shedding duration was dependent upon the initial inoculation dose.

Consistent with previous findings, Carrat and colleagues (2008b) determined that an average of 66.9 percent of influenza-inoculated participants showed clinical symptoms. Total symptom scores peaked 2 to 3 days after inoculation, and returned to baseline after 8 days. The mean duration of illness was 4.4 days (SD = 1.8 days). The curves plotted for influenza viral shedding and symptom severity were similar, with viral shedding peaking 1 day prior to clinical symptoms. However, limited information across the studies was provided on the participants who did not develop clinical illness. The authors concluded that viral shedding peaked rapidly and that symptoms for influenza-like illness varied widely, making an influenza-like illness case definition unreliable for identifying infectious individuals to implement control measures. Moreover, the study populations were adults and generally healthy. Thus, variability in age, immune status, and underlying health conditions may have profound effects on these estimates, as has been observed recently for 2009 H1N1 (Goodman, 2009). For example, children under age 9 infected with 2009 H1N1 shed virus for a median duration of 6 days after fever was detected, 1 day longer than overall median duration for all age groups, and some children showed signs of shedding for up to 13 days (Goodman, 2009).

Historically, controlled viral challenge studies have provided key insights on respiratory virus transmission (Carrat et al., 2008a). Current preliminary efforts to develop influenza voluntary challenge studies are under way in the United Kingdom and may provide an opportunity to better understand the relative contribution of differing transmission modes of influenza (Van-Tam, 2010).

A household model of transmission of pandemic 2009 H1N1 virus found an average time between symptom onset of the primary case and secondary cases to be 2.6 days (95% CI = 2.2–3.5 days), similar to previous reports of time of disease spread between household members, but shorter than the secondary infections reported below (Cauchemez et al., 2009). Another study that recruited index patients to study the serial interval of influenza leading to a secondary infection within the household found the period to be longer than previously reported: an average of 3.6 days (95% CI = 2.9–4.3 days). The interval measured time from symptom onset in a laboratory-confirmed case of influenza to the time of symptom onset in a corresponding household contact (Cowling et al., 2009b). More recently, Lau and colleagues (2010) used a community-based study of households to show that the bulk of viral shedding happened during the first 2 to 3 days after illness onset and only 1 to 8 percent of infectiousness occurs prior to symptom onset. Moreover, only 14 percent of cases that had RT-PCR–detectable influenza virus RNA were asymptomatic, and the quantity of viral particles was low among these cases, suggesting that asymptomatic cases are unlikely to play a large role in transmission.

An observational study examined influenza and rhinovirus infections among healthcare personnel. Bellei and colleagues (2007) collected both acute respiratory illness reports and laboratory samples among healthcare personnel. Nearly 50 percent of staff reporting influenza-like illnesses had rhinovirus rather than influenza. Thus, surveillance by symptoms may not accurately predict influenza viral activity among healthcare personnel. Influenza vaccination in this study population was low (19.7 percent), and varied by the department where hospital personnel were assigned. Of the 203 personnel recruited with any acute respiratory illness symptom, 48.3 percent reported direct contact with a patient, and 39.4 percent had preschool children exposure either at the hospital or at home.

Disease Transmission

In a recent study in an infant ward, of 122 susceptible patients with single rooms, only 6 (5 percent) acquired influenza in the ward, while 17 percent (13/77) of infants in a multiple-crib room acquired nosocomial infection (Hall, 2007). Overall, children with one or two roommates were nearly 4 times more likely to acquire influenza in the hospital (odds ratio = 3.90, 95% CI 2.88–4.92). The author notes that one to three separate influenza cases occurred before peak influenza activity began over the two influenza seasons that were studied, and that neither of these cases was followed by a quick outbreak in the ward. Similarly, novel data examining outbreaks of 2009 H1N1 in airplanes, buses, and schools primarily implicate close proximity transmission (Baker et al., 2010; Han et al., 2009; Kar-Purkayastha et al., 2009; Ooi et al., 2010).

In a review by Chen and colleagues (2008), transmission routes of SARS were examined. Major transmission modes that have been demonstrated include close contact via droplet spray or contaminated fomites with respiratory excretion. In addition, diarrhea accompanied infection and SARS virus was found in the greatest quantities in feces compared to nasopharyngeal and urine samples 14 days after first onset of symptoms.

Avian influenza H5N1 virus has been studied in several family clusters, and both droplet spray and contact with stool have been hypothesized as important transmission routes. In a household cluster study by Wang and colleagues (2008), an index case (the son) transmitted the infection to his father while his father cared for him in the hospital. The index case had large amounts of sputum, frequent coughing, and watery diarrhea with H5N1 infection. His father had no known exposure to poultry or other ill individuals. Neither the index case's mother nor girlfriend, both of whom also had close contact, became infected. Transmission to the father may have occurred through inhalation of respirable or inspirable particles or contact with feces-contaminated clothes. Of note, 2009 H1N1 illness symptoms also included vomiting and diarrhea (Bryant et al., 2010; Riquelme et al., 2009). Research on the potential for fecal oral transmission of 2009 H1N1 influenza is warranted.

PPE Use to Prevent Respiratory Disease Transmission

Models on the Use of PPE

The effectiveness of surgical masks and N95 respirators in reducing the spread of influenza were directly modeled as a method of preventing the 2009 H1N1 (Tracht et al., 2010). Considering that the likelihood of wearing a surgical mask or respirator can vary by many factors, including age and marital status, the authors assumed that compliance with the recommended intervention would only occur in the closed population when a minimal level of susceptible individuals became infected, and that individuals within the population could switch between wearing and not wearing masks or respirators. Several scenarios were explored, with the following results:

- when neither masks nor respirators were used, the total percentage of the population infected was estimated at 75 percent (in a population of 1 million people);
- if 10 percent of the population wore surgical masks (assumed in this scenario to be 2 percent effective in reducing susceptibility and infectivity), the total number of cases would be only minimally reduced (to approximately 73 percent);
- increasing the percentage of the population wearing surgical masks to 50 percent (assumed in this scenario to be 5 percent effective in reducing susceptibility and infectivity) reduced the infected population to approximately 69 percent;
- if 10 percent of the population wore N95 respirators (assumed in this scenario to be 20 percent effective in reducing susceptibility and infectivity), the total number of cases would be reduced to

approximately 55 percent (a reduction of approximately 19 percent from not wearing masks or respirators); and

- increasing the percentage of the population wearing N95 respirators to 50 percent (assumed in this scenario to be 50 percent effective in reducing susceptibility and infectivity) dropped the total number of cases drastically to approximately 0.1 percent.

The authors concluded that surgical masks were unlikely to impact the epidemic because of low effectiveness at reducing the spread of influenza among susceptible and infected individuals, while N95 respirators could reduce the impact of the epidemic, though they could not reduce the R_0 below 1. The authors acknowledge that the effectiveness of the interventions are time dependent and that delays in mask-use initiation can have strong effects on the findings. The results from the model suggest that healthcare personnel would benefit from widespread use of properly fitting N95 respirators among susceptible and infected individuals.

Community Studies of PPE Use

Several recent studies have looked at community use of PPE. Results of these studies have been inconsistent because of differences in study design, setting, intervention type, and ability to control for confounding factors. MacIntyre and colleagues (2009) conducted a study on the use of face masks in households in Australia during the winters of 2006 and 2007. The participating 145 households included adults with known exposure to a child with fever and other respiratory symptoms. The households were randomized to one of three arms of the trial: (1) surgical masks that were to be worn when in the same room as the ill child; (2) P2 masks (equivalent to N95 respirators), also to be worn when in the same room; and (3) a control group with no masks used. Adherence to the use of masks was found to be low (less than 50 percent). Of those who used the masks, a reduction in the risk of acquiring a respiratory infection was noted in the range of 60 to 80 percent, and no differences were seen between surgical masks and P2 masks, but the study was underpowered to determine differences between these two interventions. In addition, the authors noted that some adults may have already been in the incubation period for infection because enrollment occurred in conjunction with a sick child visit to a healthcare facility. Thus, the mask intervention may have been applied too late in the course of illness transmission within the household.

Hand hygiene has been demonstrated to provide a reduction in respiratory infections in the community setting (Aiello et al., 2008), but the role of face masks in combination with hand hygiene (i.e., layered interventions) had not been studied in a controlled intervention trial until recently. Several recent randomized community intervention studies have attempted to compare face-mask use and hand hygiene or a combination of both interventions during seasonal influenza seasons. In one study, researchers randomized university residence halls housing 1,297 student participants to use of face masks, face masks with hand hygiene, or a control group for a 6-week period during the influenza season (Aiello et al., 2010). Significant reductions in influenza-like illnesses were seen in the group using face masks and hand hygiene as compared with the control group (reductions of 35 to 51 percent after adjusting for vaccination and other factors). Compliance data were difficult to ascertain, and the mild influenza season may have impacted the results. This study provided some insights on primary prevention rather than secondary prevention of illness because the participants were asked to wear masks before influenza-like illness was observed on campus.

Larson and colleagues (2010) conducted a study examining secondary transmission of influenza infection (i.e., other than the index case) by providing one of three interventions to urban households. The 509 households were randomized to receive one of the following: (1) education on the prevention and treatment of upper respiratory infections and influenza, (2) the same educational component plus alcohol-based hand sanitizer, or (3) the educational component plus hand sanitizer and face masks (Larson et al., 2010). Compliance with wearing the face masks was low; half of the households provided with face masks reported using the face masks when they had a household member with an influenza-like illness. In multivariate analyses no differences were observed in the rate of infection.

A study by Cowling and colleagues (2009a) assessed several interventions in 259 households and used secondary transmission of laboratory-confirmed influenza infection in family members as the outcome measure. Households were identified through household members presenting to outpatient clinics with influenza-like illness confirmed as influenza A or B by rapid testing. An education intervention was provided to the 134 households in the control group, hand hygiene supplies were provided to 136 households, and 137 households received face masks and hand hygiene supplies. Data for all the households in the study found that someone in the household developed confirmed influenza in 19 percent of the households. A significant reduction in confirmed influenza was seen for households receiving an intervention within 36 hours of the onset of symptoms in the index patient; no differences were seen in a comparison of the hand hygiene and the hand hygiene plus face masks groups.

Challenges in studies of interventions in the community setting include adherence, observations for compliance, and disentangling the contribution of layered interventions (i.e., face masks and hand hygiene together) when the effect estimate size between layered and non-layered interventions may be small. Moreover, in a light influenza season difficulties in identifying cases rapidly can impact the statistical power and effectiveness of the interventions, respectively. Last, these types of studies are unable to provide insights on the modes of transmission of influenza because face masks may block both droplet spray and direct contact inoculation from hands contaminated with influenza virus.

Clinical Studies of PPE Use by Healthcare Personnel

Although the benefits of vaccination are clear (Fiore et al., 2009; Treanor et al., 1999), much less is certain about what types of respiratory PPE are needed or the value of face masks worn by healthcare personnel. Few studies have been conducted of effective PPE interventions to reduce the transmission of influenza in hospitals or other healthcare facilities to guide policy makers seeking to ensure the health and safety of healthcare personnel. The relative value of face masks versus N95 respirators in preventing influenza transmission is especially debated, and recent reviews have concluded that there are insufficient data for recommending effective PPE approaches for preventing influenza transmission (Cowling et al., 2010; Gralton and McLaws, 2010; Jefferson et al., 2010). The possible modes of transmission of influenza, the confounding variables that exist in testing alternative interventions, and the common issues inherent with study design (see Box 2-2) suggest the complexity of the problem facing both investigators and policy makers.

Several observational studies have looked at various aspects of PPE use, but usually in small numbers of healthcare personnel. Ng and colleagues (2009) performed a survey of 133 on-duty nurses, and then divided them into cases (nurses who contracted influenza-like illness during the study period) and compared them to nurses who did not. A significant difference was noted between cases and controls in use of PPE, specifically the use of gloves, gowns, and face shields. No mention was made of respiratory protection. A significant difference between the cases and controls was that cases were less likely to be vaccinated and were also more likely to have been exposed to a sick colleague without using PPE. In a survey of healthcare personnel participating in a medical mission and treating patients in crowded conditions, fewer cases of acute respiratory illness were noted for personnel using hand sanitizer; however, use of face masks was not reported to make a difference (Al-Asmary et al., 2007). A study of 32 healthcare personnel (in which one group wore face masks and the other did not) found no differences in occurrence of the common cold, but the small number of study participants did not allow for adequate exploration of the study question (Jacobs et al., 2009). A retrospective study compared "frontline" healthcare personnel confirmed to have SARS with those who did not acquire the disease (Chen et al., 2009b). The risk of contracting SARS increased for those who performed tracheal intubations of SARS patients and for those who cared for "super-spreader" SARS patients. Risk decreased for those healthcare personnel wearing multiple pairs of gloves and for those who avoided face-to-face contact with SARS patients.

Observations during the 2009 H1N1 epidemic were reported from a Singapore hospital that documented the varying requirements for respirators or face masks based on different departments of the hospital or work tasks during three phases of the 2009 H1N1 epidemic (Ang et al., 2010). No difference was seen in the transmission of H1N1 to healthcare personnel. Many healthcare personnel who were confirmed to have H1N1 had not cared for H1N1 patients and may have acquired the disease in community settings. This hospital had worked with cases of SARS in 2003, and the authors stated that adherence to PPE, although not documented, was usually strict.

Recently, the first randomized trial assessing the value of face masks compared with N95 respirators in preventing influenza among healthcare personnel was published (Loeb et al., 2009). Among the 446 nurses from 8 tertiary care hospitals in Ontario who participated in the study, 225 were assigned to wear surgical masks (the brand used at their respective hospitals), and 221 were assigned to wear N95 respirators during the 2008–2009 winter influenza season. Study participants also wore gowns and gloves (as part of routine infection control practice) when caring for patients with febrile respiratory illnesses. Online questionnaires were

---

BOX 2-2
Confounding Issues for Understanding the Transmission of
Influenza and Other Viral Respiratory Diseases

Confounding Variables in Testing Interventions
- Variability in types of and fit of mask or respirator
- Compliance with appropriate use of mask or respirator
- Measuring compliance of mask or respirator use
- Hand hygiene rates
- Levels of environmental contamination
- Duration and intensity of exposure to influenza
- Variations among patients regarding dispersal of infectious particles after cough, sneeze, normal talking
- Susceptibility of healthcare personnel (antibody titer, vaccine status)
- Community and home exposure to the virus

Issues with Study Design
- Avoiding bias
- Accounting for confounders
- Measuring all possible modes of transmission
- Study power
- Measuring infection accurately, including measuring severity (indirect measure of exposure to infecting dose)

---

used twice a week to assess symptoms of influenza. The primary outcome examined by the study was laboratory-confirmed influenza. Compliance with PPE use was determined through audits during several weeks in March and early April 2009 that were anticipated to be the peak of the influenza season. If the unit had patients with influenza or a febrile respiratory illness, auditors were sent to observe use of masks or respirators. The study stopped collecting data in late April 2009, with the reporting of novel H1N1 influenza A and the recommendation by the Ontario Ministry of Health and Long-Term Care that N95 respirators be used for caring for patients with febrile respiratory disease. Laboratory-confirmed influenza was documented in 50 of the 225 nurses allocated to wear surgical masks (23.6 percent) and in 48 of the 221 nurses allocated to wear N95 respirators (22.9 percent). The authors concluded that the similar results between groups indicated that surgical masks were noninferior to N95 respirators. Study limitations noted by the authors included challenges in assessing compliance with PPE use; lack of measurement on rates of hand hygiene or gown and glove use; and the source of infectious exposure (hospital or community exposure) could not be ascertained. Several subsequent letters to the editor noted issues including that measures of exposure risk were missing and the value of triage procedures and the adherence to cough etiquette were not measured (Srinivasan and Perl, 2009), concerns about study power (Clynes, 2010), and concerns about the lack of eye-shield protection among nurses in the study (Finkelstein et al., 2010). This study has pointed out the many challenges in assessing the effectiveness of respirators and face masks in preventing influenza transmission, including the rates of correct use and fit of respirators and masks, the level of environmental contamination, the duration and intensity of exposure, and the susceptibility of healthcare personnel to H1N1. Similar to the community intervention studies, this type of study cannot provide information on the modes of transmission of influenza in the clinical setting. In future studies, the severity of infection might be an important secondary endpoint of interest because it may reflect infectious dose. Moreover, it will be important to add higher levels of monitoring for compliance and assessment of close contacts (such as household members) to better identify sources of infection in these types of studies.

Use of Face Masks and Respirators as Source Control

Face masks and respirators have also been used as source control, that is, placing a mask on patients with respiratory illnesses in clinics or emergency departments to reduce the potential for disease transmission to other patients, family members, or healthcare personnel. Johnson and colleagues (2009) studied nine patients with documented influenza and asked each to cough 5 times into a 90 mm diameter petri dish containing transport media. With no mask on, 7 of 9 patients had detectable virus. However, with either a surgical mask or N95 mask on, no virus was detected. The authors concluded that as a source control, masks were equally effective in preventing dissemination. Because this was not a study of transmission, however, one can only say that the concept of droplet spray dissemination being controlled with a surgical mask is plausible, but unconfirmed.

SUMMARY OF PROGRESS

Animal studies have found that the ferret and guinea pig models appear to be highly representative of humans in terms of their susceptibility to infection, the influenza viral strains that display a transmissible phenotype, and the kinetics with which transmission occurs. Experiments performed in both of these animal models suggest that transmission of influenza viruses can proceed by both droplet spray as well as aerosol modes, which would include respirable particles. Animal studies have also pointed to a number of environmental factors, including relative humidity and temperature that may influence transmission. Recent studies that have employed environmental monitoring of the air for influenza, as well as others that have examined contamination of fomites and hands with H1N1, have provided insights on the potential for influenza-virus contamination of the healthcare environment. Nonetheless, data on the viability of influenza in air samples and fomites in these settings are limited. Mathematical models have been developed to better characterize the relative contribution of influenza transmission modes. Available, well-specified parameters for these models are limited because information is lacking on the viability of influenza in aerosols, salivary virus concentrations, amounts of virus in respirable and inspirable particles, and the quantity and persistence of viability on various fomites in the healthcare setting. Taken together, progress has been made in understanding the modes of transmission, but the relative contributions of the modes are still unclear. Much remains to be learned about the effectiveness of control measures to prevent transmission.

Observational studies and controlled studies relevant to PPE use and transmission of influenza or other viral respiratory diseases are limited because study protocols were largely not in place for 2009 H1N1 or for recent seasonal flu periods, and studies have not provided adequate power to answer questions regarding the effectiveness of using PPE in reducing or preventing disease transmission.

FINDINGS AND RESEARCH NEEDS

As discussed throughout this chapter, much remains to be learned about the transmission of influenza and other viral respiratory diseases. The committee's overall findings in this area (Box 2-3) highlight the current limitations on data regarding transmission that are needed to inform decisions on the protection of healthcare personnel and patients. The committee heard about a number of ongoing research efforts at its June 2010 workshop (Appendix A). Sustained efforts will be critical, as prior research efforts from the 1940s to 1990s have largely ebbed between pandemics.

The committee has identified a range of research efforts, some of which can be addressed expeditiously (in the next 6 to 12 months) and have a significant impact on improving the nation's readiness for pandemic influenza; long-term studies are also needed to more fully understand disease transmission and prevention strategies. As in the 2008 IOM report, the recommendations focus on a comprehensive research strategy to address critical questions in as expedited and coordinated manner as possible.

BOX 2-3
Findings

- Standardized terms, definitions, and appropriate classifications are needed to properly describe transmission routes and aerodynamic diameter of particles associated with respiratory disease transmission.
- Influenza and other respiratory viruses differ in virulence and transmission routes.
- A comprehensive research strategy is needed. Transmission routes need to be better understood to select appropriate personal protective equipment (PPE) and better protect healthcare personnel and patients. An in-depth understanding of the relative contribution of the transmission routes will require research at many levels, including basic science laboratory studies, monitoring studies, environmental intervention studies, and clinical and community-based studies.
- To determine the risk of specific exposures and tasks, research should be done to characterize the aerodynamic diameter of particles and concentration of influenza in aerosols generated by various procedures to enable a comparison of aerosol sizes and concentrations of influenza generated by coughing, sneezing, talking, and exhalation.
- The potential for confounding and complexity in conducting intervention studies of the effectiveness of PPE within the clinical setting makes it impossible to determine various routes of transmission in this setting. Instead, clinical intervention and observational studies of PPE will continue to be useful in determining the effectiveness of disease prevention measures albeit without a complete understanding of the specific mechanisms and to garner information on the best precautionary measures for future outbreaks of influenza or other viral respiratory diseases.
- Little is known about the potential PPE role of face shields and face masks in preventing transmission of viral respiratory diseases.

Animal studies Although data in ferrets and guinea pigs indicate that vaccination, antiviral treatment, and altered environmental conditions can each reduce or abrogate transmission, confirmatory and more in-depth experimentation would be valuable in determining which interventions are likely to be the most effective. In vivo studies on the impacts of increased air exchange and UV treatment of air would also be highly informative and relatively simple to execute in an animal model.

Environmental studies Future studies are needed to assess whether the identified influenza RNA in aerosol samplers (in multiple locations, e.g., schools, trains, healthcare facilities) are viable and reflect the extent to which individuals are exposed to aerosols of influenza within these environments. In addition, the impact of environmental factors, such as UV and humidity, on influenza transmission and infection should be examined in the community and healthcare setting.

Modeling studies Statistical and mathematical models need to be evaluated for their utility in prediction and inferences regarding the relative contributions of different transmission modes in varying environmental/community contexts. Collaborations between experimental or observational research and mathematical modelers are warranted so that the parameters used in mathematical models are based on rigorous data and provide evidence that would help narrow parameter estimates used in modeling.

Clinical studies Appropriately powered studies are needed that examine all possible modes of transmission, measure the rates of compliance with each intervention of interest, and define the pre-exposure influenza antibody titers of study subjects. Environmental levels of contamination need to be studied, including cultures from air sampling and swabs of hard surfaces. Serological studies of exposure to influenza virus in family members or roommates would be a reasonable marker of home exposure during the study period. Useful measures would also include the distribution of the size of respiratory particles of patients exposed to the healthcare personnel and some measure of the intensity of the exposure to patients that might include distance from, time in contact with, and specific procedures performed on the infected patients.

Studies on the role of PPE The potential role of face shields and face masks as PPE should be explored to determine the level of protection from droplet spray transmission. The role of fomites is unclear in the healthcare setting. Additional studies are needed to determine what role gowns, gloves, face masks, and respirators might play in influenza transmission. Further work on donning and doffing processes is also needed. Studies should examine whether antiviral-coated PPE provides any additional protection and how maintenance and reuse are affected.

RECOMMENDATIONS

Recommendation: Develop Standardized Terms and Definitions
CDC and the Occupational Safety and Health Administration, in partnership with other relevant agencies and organizations, should work to develop standardized terms, definitions, and appropriate classifications to describe transmission routes and aerodynamic diameter of particles associated with viral respiratory disease transmission. This effort should involve a consensus from the industrial hygiene, infectious disease, and healthcare communities.

Recommendation: Develop and Implement a Comprehensive Research Strategy to Understand Viral Respiratory Disease Transmission
The National Institutes of Health, in collaboration with other research agencies and organizations, should develop and fund a comprehensive research strategy to improve the understanding of viral respiratory disease transmission, including, but not limited to, examining the characteristics of influenza transmission, animal models, human challenge studies, and intervention trials. This strategy should include

- **an expedited mechanism for funding these types of studies and**
- **clinical research centers of excellence for studying influenza and other respiratory virus transmission.**

REFERENCES

Aiello, A. E., R. M. Coulborn, V. Perez, and E. L. Larson. 2008. Effect of hand hygiene on infectious disease risk in the community setting: A meta-analysis. *American Journal of Public Health* 98(8):1372-1381.

Aiello, A. E., G. F. Murray, V. Perez, R. M. Coulborn, B. M. Davis, M. Uddin, D. K. Shay, S. H. Waterman, and A. S. Monto. 2010. Mask use, hand hygiene, and seasonal influenza-like illness among young adults: A randomized intervention trial. *Journal of Infectious Diseases* 201(4):491-498.

Al-Asmary, S., A. S. Al-Shehri, A. Abou-Zeid, M. Abdel-Fattah, T. Hifnawy, and T. El-Said. 2007. Acute respiratory tract infections among Hajj medical mission personnel, Saudi Arabia. *International Journal of Infectious Diseases* 11(3):268-272.

Alford, R. H., J. A. Kasel, P. J. Gerone, and V. Knight. 1966. Human influenza resulting from aerosol inhalation. *Proceedings of the Society for Experimental Biology and Medicine* 122(3):800-804.

Ali, M. J., C. Z. Teh, R. Jennings, and C. W. Potter. 1982. Transmissibility of influenza viruses in hamsters. *Archives of Virology* 72(3):187-197.

Andrewes, C. H., and R. E. Glover. 1941. Spread of infection from the respiratory tract of the ferret. I. Transmission of influenza A virus. *British Journal of Experimental Pathology* 22:91-97.

Ang, B., B. F. Poh, M. K. Win, and A. Chow. 2010. Surgical masks for protection of health care personnel against pandemic novel swine-origin influenza A (H1N1)-2009: Results from an observational study. *Clinical Infectious Diseases* 50(7):1011-1014.

Atkinson, M. P., and L. M. Wein. 2008. Quantifying the routes of transmission for pandemic influenza. *Bulletin of Mathematical Biology* 70(3):820-867.

Baker, M. G., C. N. Thornley, C. Mills, S. Roberts, S. Perera, J. Peters, A. Kelso, I. Barr, and N. Wilson. 2010. Transmission of pandemic A/H1N1 2009 influenza on passenger aircraft: Retrospective cohort study. *British Medical Journal* 340:c2424.

Bellei, N., E. Carraro, A. H. S. Perosa, D. Benfica, and C. F. H. Granato. 2007. Influenza and rhinovirus infections among health-care workers. *Respirology* 12(1):100-103.

Belser, J. A., O. Blixt, L. M. Chen, C. Pappas, T. R. Maines, N. Van Hoeven, R. Donis, J. Busch, R. McBride, J. C. Paulson, J. M. Katz, and T. M. Tumpey. 2008. Contemporary North American influenza H7 viruses possess human receptor specificity: Implications for virus transmissibility. *Proceedings of the National Academy of Sciences (U.S.A.)* 105(21):7558-7563.

Blachere, F. M., W. G. Lindsley, T. A. Pearce, S. E. Anderson, M. Fisher, R. Khakoo, B. J. Meade, O. Lander, S. Davis, R. E. Thewlis, I. Celik, B. T. Chen, and D. H. Beezhold. 2009. Measurement of airborne influenza virus in a hospital emergency department. *Clinical Infectious Diseases* 48(4):438-440.

Boone, S. A., and C. P. Gerba. 2007. Significance of fomites in the spread of respiratory and enteric viral disease. *Applied and Environmental Microbiology* 73(6):1687-1696.

Brankston, G., L. Gitterman, Z. Hirji, C. Lemieux, and M. Gardam. 2007. Transmission of influenza A in human beings. *Lancet Infectious Diseases* 7(4):257-265.

Brauer, F. 2009. Mathematical epidemiology is not an oxymoron. *BMC Public Health* 9(Suppl. 1):S2.

Bryant, P. A., M. Tebruegge, G. Papadakis, C. Clarke, P. Barnett, A. J. Daley, M. South, and N. Curtis. 2010. Clinical and microbiologic features associated with novel swine-origin influenza A pandemic 2009 (H1N1) virus in children: A prospective cohort study. *Pediatric Infectious Disease Journal* 29(8):694-698.

Carrat, F., E. Vergu, N. M. Ferguson, M. Lemaitre, S. Cauchemez, S. Leach, and A. J. Valleron. 2008a. Time lines of infection and disease in human influenza: A review of volunteer challenge studies. *American Journal of Epidemiology* 167(7):775-785.

———. 2008b. Time lines of infection and disease in human influenza: A review of volunteer challenge studies. *American Journal of Epidemiology* 167(7):775-785.

Casanova, L., W. A. Rutala, D. J. Weber, and M. D. Sobsey. 2010. Coronavirus survival on healthcare personal protective equipment. *Infection Control and Hospital Epidemiology* 31(5):560-561.

Cauchemez, S., C. A. Donnelly, C. Reed, A. C. Ghani, C. Fraser, C. K. Kent, L. Finelli, and N. M. Ferguson. 2009. Household transmission of 2009 pandemic influenza A (H1N1) virus in the United States. *New England Journal of Medicine* 361(27):2619-2627.

Chen, S. C., C. P. Chio, L. J. Jou, and C. M. Liao. 2009a. Viral kinetics and exhaled droplet size affect indoor transmission dynamics of influenza infection. *Indoor Air* 19(5):401-413.

Chen, W. Q., W. H. Ling, C. Y. Lu, Y. T. Hao, Z. N. Lin, L. Ling, J. Huang, G. Li, and G. M. Yan. 2009b. Which preventive measures might protect health care workers from SARS? *BMC Public Health* 9:81.

Chen, Y.-C., S.-C. Chang, K.-S. Tsai, and F.-Y. Lin. 2008. Certainties and uncertainties facing emerging respiratory infectious diseases: Lessons from SARS. *Journal of the Formosan Medical Association* 107(6):432-442.

Clynes, N. 2010. Surgical masks vs. N95 respirators for preventing influenza. *Journal of the American Medical Association* 303(10):937-938; author reply 938-939.

Couch, R. B., R. G. Douglas, Jr., D. S. Fedson, and J. A. Kasel. 1971. Correlated studies of a recombinant influenza-virus vaccine. 3. Protection against experimental influenza in man. *Journal of Infectious Diseases* 124(5):473-480.

Couch, R. B., J. A. Kasel, J. L. Gerin, J. L. Schulman, and E. D. Kilbourne. 1974. Induction of partial immunity to influenza by a neuraminidase-specific vaccine. *Journal of Infectious Diseases* 129(4):411-420.

Cowling, B. J., K.-H. Chan, V. J. Fang, C. K. Y. Cheng, R. O. P. Fung, W. Wai, J. Sin, W. H. Seto, R. Yung, D. W. S. Chu, B. C. F. Chiu, P. W. Y. Lee, M. C. Chiu, H. C. Lee, T. M. Uyeki, P. M. Houck, J. S. M. Peiris, and G. M. Leung. 2009a. Facemasks and hand hygiene to prevent influenza transmission in households: A cluster randomized trial. *Annals of Internal Medicine* 151(7):437-446.

Cowling, B. J., V. J. Fang, S. Riley, J. S. Malik Peiris, and G. M. Leung. 2009b. Estimation of the serial interval of influenza. *Epidemiology* 20(3):344-347.

Cowling, B. J., Y. Zhou, D. K. Ip, G. M. Leung, and A. E. Aiello. 2010. Face masks to prevent transmission of influenza virus: A systematic review. *Epidemiology and Infection* 138(4):449-456.

Cunney, R. J., A. Bialachowski, D. Thornley, F. M. Smaill, and R. A. Pennie. 2000. An outbreak of influenza A in a neonatal intensive care unit. *Infection Control and Hospital Epidemiology* 21(7):449-454.

Douglas, R. G. 1975. Influenza in man. In *The influenza viruses and influenza*, edited by E. Kilbourne. New York: Academic Press. Pp. 395-447.

Drinka, P. J., P. Krause, M. Schilling, B. A. Miller, P. Shult, and S. Gravenstein. 1996. Report of an outbreak: Nursing home architecture and influenza-A attack rates. *Journal of the American Geriatrics Society* 44(8):910-913.

Drinka, P. J., P. Krause, L. Nest, and D. Tyndall. 2004. Report of an outbreak: Nursing home architecture and influenza-A attack rates: Update. *Journal of the American Geriatrics Society* 52(5):847-848.

Fabian, P., J. J. McDevitt, W. H. DeHaan, R. O. P. Fung, B. J. Cowling, K. H. Chan, G. M. Leung, and D. K. Milton. 2008. Influenza virus in human exhaled breath: An observational study. *PLoS ONE* 3(7):e2691.

Finkelstein, Y., T. Schechter, and S. B. Freedman. 2010. Surgical masks vs. N95 respirators for preventing influenza. *Journal of the American Medical Association* 303(10):938; author reply 938-939.

Fiore, A. E., C. B. Bridges, and N. J. Cox. 2009. Seasonal influenza vaccines. *Current Topics in Microbiology and Immunology* 333:43-82.

Fowler, R. A., C. B. Guest, S. E. Lapinsky, W. J. Sibbald, M. Louie, P. Tang, A. E. Simor, and T. E. Stewart. 2004. Transmission of severe acute respiratory syndrome during intubation and mechanical ventilation. *American Journal of Respiratory and Critical Care Medicine* 169(11):1198-1202.

Francis, T., and T. P. Magill. 1935. Immunological studies with the virus of influenza. *Journal of Experimental Medicine* 62(4):505-516.

Furuya, H. 2007. Risk of transmission of airborne infection during train commute based on mathematical model. *Environmental Health and Preventive Medicine* 12(2):78-83.

Gao, Y., Y. Zhang, K. Shinya, G. Deng, Y. Jiang, Z. Li, Y. Guan, G. Tian, Y. Li, J. Shi, L. Liu, X. Zeng, Z. Bu, X. Xia, Y. Kawaoka, and H. Chen. 2009. Identification of amino acids in HA and PB2 critical for the transmission of H5N1 avian influenza viruses in a mammalian host. *PLoS Pathogens* 5(12):e1000709.

Goodman, A. 2009. *Viral shedding prolonged in children with H1N1 flu, especially younger children.* http://www.medscape.com/viewarticle/711619 (accessed December 8, 2010).

Gralton, J., and M. L. McLaws. 2010. Protecting healthcare workers from pandemic influenza: N95 or surgical masks? *Critical Care Medicine* 38(2):657-667.

Gregg, M. B. 1980. The epidemiology of influenza in humans. *Annals of the New York Academy of Sciences* 353:45-53.

Gwaltney, J. M., Jr., P. B. Moskalski, and J. O. Hendley. 1978. Hand-to-hand transmission of rhinovirus colds. *Annals of Internal Medicine* 88(4):463-467.

Hall, C. B. 2007. The spread of influenza and other respiratory viruses: Complexities and conjectures. *Clinical Infectious Diseases* 45(3):353-359.

Hall, C. B., R. G. Douglas, Jr., and J. M. Geiman. 1980. Possible transmission by fomites of respiratory syncytial virus. *Journal of Infectious Diseases* 141(1):98-102.

Hall, C. B., R. G. Douglas, Jr., K. C. Schnabel, and J. M. Geiman. 1981. Infectivity of respiratory syncytial virus by various routes of inoculation. *Infection and Immunity* 33(3):779-783.

Halloran, M. E., F. G. Hayden, Y. Yang, I. M. Longini, Jr., and A. S. Monto. 2007. Antiviral effects on influenza viral transmission and pathogenicity: Observations from household-based trials. *American Journal of Epidemiology* 165(2):212-221.

Han, K., X. Zhu, F. He, L. Liu, L. Zhang, H. Ma, X. Tang, T. Huang, G. Zeng, and B. P. Zhu. 2009. Lack of airborne transmission during outbreak of pandemic (H1N1) 2009 among tour group members, China, June 2009. *Emerging Infectious Diseases* 15(10):1578-1581.

Harper, G. J. 1961. Airborne micro-organisms: Survival tests with four viruses. *Journal of Hygiene (London)* 59:479-486.

———. 1963. The influence of environment on the survival of airborne virus particles in the laboratory. *Archiv für die Gesamte Virusforschung* 13:64-71.

Hayden, F. G., L. V. Gubareva, A. S. Monto, T. C. Klein, M. J. Elliot, J. M. Hammond, S. J. Sharp, and M. J. Ossi. 2000. Inhaled zanamivir for the prevention of influenza in families. Zanamivir family study group. *New England Journal of Medicine* 343(18):1282-1289.

Hayden, F. G., R. Belshe, C. Villanueva, R. Lanno, C. Hughes, I. Small, R. Dutkowski, P. Ward, and J. Carr. 2004. Management of influenza in households: A prospective, randomized comparison of oseltamivir treatment with or without postexposure prophylaxis. *Journal of Infectious Diseases* 189(3):440-449.

Hemmes, J. H., K. C. Winkler, and S. M. Kool. 1960. Virus survival as a seasonal factor in influenza and polimyelitis. *Nature* 188:430-431.

Hendley, J. O., R. P. Wenzel, and J. M. Gwaltney, Jr. 1973. Transmission of rhinovirus colds by self-inoculation. *New England Journal of Medicine* 288(26):1361-1364.

Hsu, S. B., and Y. H. Hsieh. 2008. On the role of asymptomatic infection in transmission dynamics of infectious diseases. *Bulletin of Mathematical Biology* 70(1):134-155.

IOM (Institute of Medicine). 2008. *Preparing for an influenza pandemic: Personal protective equipment for healthcare workers.* Washington, DC: The National Academies Press.

Itoh, Y., K. Shinya, M. Kiso, T. Watanabe, Y. Sakoda, M. Hatta, Y. Muramoto, D. Tamura, Y. Sakai-Tagawa, T. Noda, S. Sakabe, M. Imai, Y. Hatta, S. Watanabe, C. Li, S. Yamada, K. Fujii, S. Murakami, H. Imai, S. Kakugawa, M. Ito, R. Takano, K. Iwatsuki-Horimoto, M. Shimojima, T. Horimoto, H. Goto, K. Takahashi, A. Makino, H. Ishigaki, M. Nakayama, M. Okamatsu, D. Warshauer, P. A. Shult, R. Saito, H. Suzuki, Y. Furuta, M. Yamashita, K. Mitamura, K. Nakano, M. Nakamura, R. Brockman-Schneider, H. Mitamura, M. Yamazaki, N. Sugaya, M. Suresh, M. Ozawa, G. Neumann, J. Gern, H. Kida, K. Ogasawara, and Y. Kawaoka. 2009. In vitro and in vivo characterization of new swine-origin H1N1 influenza viruses. *Nature* 460(7258):1021-1025.

Jacobs, J. L., S. Ohde, O. Takahashi, Y. Tokuda, F. Omata, and T. Fukui. 2009. Use of surgical face masks to reduce the incidence of the common cold among health care workers in Japan: A randomized controlled trial. *American Journal of Infection Control* 37(5):417-419.

Jefferson, T., C. Del Mar, L. Dooley, E. Ferroni, L. A. Al-Ansary, G. A. Bawazeer, M. L. van Driel, S. Nair, R. Foxlee, and A. Rivetti. 2010. Physical interventions to interrupt or reduce the spread of respiratory viruses. *Cochrane Database of Systematic Reviews* 1:CD006207.

Johnson, D. F., J. D. Druce, C. Birch, and M. L. Grayson. 2009. A quantitative assessment of the efficacy of surgical and N95 masks to filter influenza virus in patients with acute influenza infection. *Clinical Infectious Diseases* 49(2):275-277.

Kar-Purkayastha, I., C. Ingram, H. Maguire, and A. Roche. 2009. The importance of school and social activities in the transmission of influenza A(H1N1)v: England, April-June 2009. *Euro Surveillance* 14(33).

Klontz, K. C., N. A. Hynes, R. A. Gunn, M. H. Wilder, M. W. Harmon, and A. P. Kendal. 1989. An outbreak of influenza A/Taiwan/1/86 (H1N1) infections at a naval base and its association with airplane travel. *American Journal of Epidemiology* 129(2):341-348.

Larson, E. L., Y. H. Ferng, J. Wong-McLoughlin, S. Wang, M. Haber, and S. S. Morse. 2010. Impact of non-pharmaceutical interventions on URIs and influenza in crowded, urban households. *Public Health Reports* 125(2):178-191.

Lau, L. L., B. J. Cowling, V. J. Fang, K. H. Chan, E. H. Lau, M. Lipsitch, C. K. Cheng, P. M. Houck, T. M. Uyeki, J. S. Peiris, and G. M. Leung. 2010. Viral shedding and clinical illness in naturally acquired influenza virus infections. *Journal of Infectious Diseases* 201(10):1509-1516.

Li, Y., P. Leung, L. Yao, Q. W. Song, and E. Newton. 2006. Antimicrobial effect of surgical masks coated with nanoparticles. *Journal of Hospital Infection* 62(1):58-63.

Lindsley, W. G., F. M. Blachere, K. A. Davis, T. A. Pearce, M. A. Fisher, R. Khakoo, S. M. Davis, M. E. Rogers, R. E. Thewlis, J. A. Posada, J. B. Redrow, I. B. Celik, B. T. Chen, and D. H. Beezhold. 2010a. Distribution of airborne influenza virus and respiratory syncytial virus in an urgent care medical clinic. *Clinical Infectious Diseases* 50(5):693-698.

Lindsley, W. G., F. M. Blachere, R. E. Thewlis, A. Vishnu, K. A. Davis, G. Cao, J. E. Palmer, K. E. Clark, M. A. Fisher, R. Khakoo, and D. H. Beezhold. 2010b. Measurements of airborne influenza virus in aerosol particles from human coughs. *PLoS ONE [Electronic Resource]* 5(11):e15100.

Loeb, M., A. McGeer, B. Henry, M. Ofner, D. Rose, T. Hlywka, J. Levie, J. McQueen, S. Smith, L. Moss, A. Smith, K. Green, and S. D. Walter. 2004. SARS among critical care nurses, Toronto. *Emerging Infectious Diseases* 10(2):251-255.

Loeb, M., N. Dafoe, J. Mahony, M. John, A. Sarabia, V. Glavin, R. Webby, M. Smieja, D. J. D. Earn, S. Chong, A. Webb, and S. D. Walter. 2009. Surgical mask vs. N95 respirator for preventing influenza among health care workers a randomized trial. *Journal of the American Medical Association* 302(17):1865-1871.

Lowen, A., and P. Palese. 2009. Transmission of influenza virus in temperate zones is predominantly by aerosol, in the tropics by contact: A hypothesis. *PLoS Currents Influenza* 1:RRN1002.

Lowen, A. C., S. Mubareka, T. M. Tumpey, A. Garcia-Sastre, and P. Palese. 2006. The guinea pig as a transmission model for human influenza viruses. *Proceedings of the National Academy of Sciences (U.S.A.)* 103(26):9988-9992.

Lowen, A. C., S. Mubareka, J. Steel, and P. Palese. 2007. Influenza virus transmission is dependent on relative humidity and temperature. *PLoS Pathogens* 3(10):1470-1476.

Lowen, A. C., J. Steel, S. Mubareka, and P. Palese. 2008. High temperature (30 degrees C) blocks aerosol but not contact transmission of influenza virus. *Journal of Virology* 82(11):5650-5652.

Lowen, A. C., J. Steel, S. Mubareka, E. Carnero, A. Garcia-Sastre, and P. Palese. 2009. Blocking interhost transmission of influenza virus by vaccination in the guinea pig model. *Journal of Virology* 83(7):2803-2818.

Macias, A. E., A. de la Torre, S. Moreno-Espinosa, P. E. Leal, M. T. Bourlon, and G. M. Ruiz-Palacios. 2009. Controlling the novel A (H1N1) influenza virus: Don't touch your face! *Journal of Hospital Infection* 73(3):280-281.

MacIntyre, C. R., S. Cauchemez, D. E. Dwyer, H. Seale, P. Cheung, G. Browne, M. Fasher, J. Wood, Z. Gao, R. Booy, and N. Ferguson. 2009. Face mask use and control of respiratory virus transmission in households. *Emerging Infectious Diseases* 15(2):233-241.

Maines, T. R., L. M. Chen, Y. Matsuoka, H. Chen, T. Rowe, J. Ortin, A. Falcon, T. H. Nguyen, Q. Mai le, E. R. Sedyaningsih, S. Harun, T. M. Tumpey, R. O. Donis, N. J. Cox, K. Subbarao, and J. M. Katz. 2006. Lack of transmission of H5N1 avian-human reassortant influenza viruses in a ferret model. *Proceedings of the National Academy of Sciences (U.S.A.)* 103(32):12121-12126.

Maines, T. R., A. Jayaraman, J. A. Belser, D. A. Wadford, C. Pappas, H. Zeng, K. M. Gustin, M. B. Pearce, K. Viswanathan, Z. H. Shriver, R. Raman, N. J. Cox, R. Sasisekharan, J. M. Katz, and T. M. Tumpey. 2009. Transmission and pathogenesis of swine-origin 2009 A(H1N1) influenza viruses in ferrets and mice. *Science* 325(5939):484-487.

Mitchell, C. A., and L. F. Guerin. 1972. Influenza A of human, swine, equine and avian origin: Comparison of survival in aerosol form. *Canadian Journal of Comparative Medicine* 36(1):9-11.

Mitchell, C. A., L. F. Guerin, and J. Robillard. 1968. Decay of influenza A viruses of human and avian origin. *Canadian Journal of Comparative Medicine* 32(4):544-546.

Monto, A. S., M. E. Pichichero, S. J. Blanckenberg, O. Ruuskanen, C. Cooper, D. M. Fleming, and C. Kerr. 2002. Zanamivir prophylaxis: An effective strategy for the prevention of influenza types A and B within households. *Journal of Infectious Diseases* 186(11):1582-1588.

Morens, D. M., and V. M. Rash. 1995. Lessons from a nursing home outbreak of influenza A. *Infection Control and Hospital Epidemiology* 16(5):275-280.

Moser, M. R., T. R. Bender, H. S. Margolis, G. R. Noble, A. P. Kendal, and D. G. Ritter. 1979. An outbreak of influenza aboard a commercial airliner. *American Journal of Epidemiology* 110(1):1-6.

Mubareka, S., A. C. Lowen, J. Steel, A. L. Coates, A. Garcia-Sastre, and P. Palese. 2009. Transmission of influenza virus via aerosols and fomites in the guinea pig model. *Journal of Infectious Diseases* 199(6):858-865.

Munster, V. J., E. de Wit, J. M. A. van den Brand, S. Herfst, E. J. A. Schrauwen, T. M. Bestebroer, D. van de Vijver, C. A. Boucher, M. Koopmans, G. F. Rimmelzwaan, T. Kuiken, A. Osterhaus, and R. A. M. Fouchier. 2009. Pathogenesis and transmission of swine-origin 2009 A(H1N1) influenza virus in ferrets. *Science* 325(5939):481-483.

Ng, T. C., N. Lee, S. C. Hui, R. Lai, and M. Ip. 2009. Preventing healthcare workers from acquiring influenza. *Infection Control and Hospital Epidemiology* 30(3):292-295.

Nicas, M., and R. M. Jones. 2009. Relative contributions of four exposure pathways to influenza infection risk. *Risk Analysis* 29(9):1292-1303.

Nicas, M., and G. Sun. 2006. An integrated model of infection risk in a health-care environment. *Risk Analysis* 26(4):1085-1096.

Ooi, P. L., F. Y. Lai, C. L. Low, R. Lin, C. Wong, M. Hibberd, and P. A. Tambyah. 2010. Clinical and molecular evidence for transmission of novel influenza A(H1N1/2009) on a commercial airplane. *Archives of Internal Medicine* 170(10):913-915.

Riquelme, A., M. Alvarez-Lobos, C. Pavez, P. Hasbun, J. Dabanch, C. Cofre, J. Jimenez, and M. Calvo. 2009. Gastrointestinal manifestations among chilean patients infected with novel influenza A (H1N1) 2009 virus. *Gut* 58(11):1567-1568.

Schaffer, F. L., M. E. Soergel, and D. C. Straube. 1976. Survival of airborne influenza virus: Effects of propagating host, relative humidity, and composition of spray fluids. *Archives of Virology* 51(4):263-273.

Schulman, J. L. 1967. Experimental transmission of influenza virus infection in mice. IV. Relationship of transmissibility of different strains of virus and recovery of airborne virus in the environment of infector mice. *Journal of Experimental Medicine* 125(3):479-488.

———. 1968. The use of an animal model to study transmission of influenza virus infection. *American Journal of Public Health and the Nation's Health* 58(11):2092-2096.

Schulman, J. I., and E. D. Kilbourne. 1962. Airborne transmission of influenza virus infection in mice. *Nature* 195:1129-1130.

Shaman, J., V. E. Pitzer, C. Viboud, B. T. Grenfell, and M. Lipsitch. 2010. Absolute humidity and the seasonal onset of influenza in the continental United States. *PLoS Biology* 8(2):e1000316.

Smith, W., C. H. Andrewes, and P. P. Laidlaw. 1933. A virus obtained from influenza patients. *Lancet* 8:66-68.

Sorrell, E. M., H. Wan, Y. Araya, H. Song, and D. R. Perez. 2009. Minimal molecular constraints for respiratory droplet transmission of an avian-human H9N2 influenza A virus. *Proceedings of the National Academy of Sciences (U.S.A.)* 106(18):7565-7570.

Srinivasan, A., and T. M. Perl. 2009. Respiratory protection against influenza. *Journal of the American Medical Association* 302(17):1903-1904.

Steel, J., A. C. Lowen, S. Mubareka, and P. Palese. 2009. Transmission of influenza virus in a mammalian host is increased by PB2 amino acids 627K or 627E/701N. *PLoS Pathogens* 5(1):e1000252.

Steel, J., P. Staeheli, S. Mubareka, A. Garcia-Sastre, P. Palese, and A. C. Lowen. 2010. Transmission of pandemic H1N1 influenza virus and impact of prior exposure to seasonal strains or interferon treatment. *Journal of Virology* 84(1):21-26.

Tellier, R. 2009. Aerosol transmission of influenza A virus: A review of new studies. *Journal of the Royal Society Interface* 6(Suppl. 6):S783-S790.

Tracht, S. M., S. Y. Del Valle, and J. M. Hyman. 2010. Mathematical modeling of the effectiveness of facemasks in reducing the spread of novel influenza A (H1N1). *PLoS ONE* 5(2):e9018.

Treanor, J. J., K. Kotloff, R. F. Betts, R. Belshe, F. Newman, D. Iacuzio, J. Wittes, and M. Bryant. 1999. Evaluation of trivalent, live, cold-adapted (CAIV-T) and inactivated (TIV) influenza vaccines in prevention of virus infection and illness following challenge of adults with wild-type influenza A (H1N1), A (H3N2), and B viruses. *Vaccine* 18(9-10):899-906.

Tumpey, T. M., T. R. Maines, N. Van Hoeven, L. Glaser, A. Solorzano, C. Pappas, N. J. Cox, D. E. Swayne, P. Palese, J. M. Katz, and A. Garcia-Sastre. 2007. A two-amino acid change in the hemagglutinin of the 1918 influenza virus abolishes transmission. *Science* 315(5812):655-659.

Van Hoeven, N., C. Pappas, J. A. Belser, T. R. Maines, H. Zeng, A. Garcia-Sastre, R. Sasisekharan, J. M. Katz, and T. M. Tumpey. 2009. Human HA and polymerase subunit PB2 proteins confer transmission of an avian influenza virus through the air. *Proceedings of the National Academy of Sciences (U.S.A.)* 106(9):3366-3371.

Van-Tam, J. 2010. *Update on influenza challenge studies in the UK.* Presentation at the Institute of Medicine workshop on Current Research Issues—Personal Protective Equipment for Healthcare Workers to Prevent Transmission of Pandemic Influenza and Other Viral Respiratory Infections, June 3, Washington, DC. http://iom.edu/~/media/Files/Activity% 20Files/PublicHealth/PPECurrentResearch/2010-JUN-3/Van%20Tam%20% 20Panel%201%20approved%20for%20web.pdf (accessed December 8, 2010).

Wan, H., E. M. Sorrell, H. Song, M. J. Hossain, G. Ramirez-Nieto, I. Monne, J. Stevens, G. Cattoli, I. Capua, L. M. Chen, R. O. Donis, J. Busch, J. C. Paulson, C. Brockwell, R. Webby, J. Blanco, M. Q. Al-Natour, and D. R. Perez. 2008. Replication and transmission of H9N2 influenza viruses in ferrets: Evaluation of pandemic potential. *PLoS ONE* 3(8):e2923.

Wang, H., Z. Feng, Y. Shu, H. Yu, L. Zhou, R. Zu, Y. Huai, J. Dong, C. Bao, L. Wen, H. Wang, P. Yang, W. Zhao, L. Dong, M. Zhou, Q. Liao, H. Yang, M. Wang, X. Lu, Z. Shi, W. Wang, L. Gu, F. Zhu, Q. Li, W. Yin, W. Yang, D. Li, T. M. Uyeki, and Y. Wang. 2008. Probable limited person-to-person transmission of highly pathogenic avian influenza A (H5N1) virus in China. *Lancet* 371(9622):1427-1434.

Weber, T. P., and N. I. Stilianakis. 2008. Inactivation of influenza A viruses in the environment and modes of transmission: A critical review. *Journal of Infection* 57(5):361-373.

Welliver, R., A. S. Monto, O. Carewicz, E. Schatteman, M. Hassman, J. Hedrick, H. C. Jackson, L. Huson, P. Ward, and J. S. Oxford. 2001. Effectiveness of oseltamivir in preventing influenza in household contacts: A randomized controlled trial. *Journal of the American Medical Association* 285(6):748-754.

Wong, B. C., N. Lee, Y. Li, P. K. Chan, H. Qiu, Z. Luo, R. W. Lai, K. L. Ngai, D. S. Hui, K. W. Choi, and I. T. Yu. 2010. Possible role of aerosol transmission in a hospital outbreak of influenza. *Clinical Infectious Diseases* 51(10):1176-1183.

3

Designing and Engineering Effective PPE

Understanding workplace hazards is critically important to ensuring that personal protective equipment (PPE) is available to healthcare personnel facing an influenza pandemic or other hazardous working conditions. Research on the transmission and virulence of the influenza virus and other potential infectious agents (Chapter 2) will inform decisions on the design and engineering of healthcare PPE.

As innovative approaches begin to address the PPE challenges of the healthcare workplace, further efforts are needed that focus on how to address the unique or varied issues that healthcare personnel face—easy communications with patients and families, PPE that can be changed or reused between different patients, PPE that is comfortable during long wear times, and PPE that does not interfere with work performance. Healthcare personnel are not alone in having job-specific PPE requirements. Firefighters need PPE that addresses high temperatures, construction workers on roofs and high-rise structures need protection from falls, and both have many other PPE requirements. Innovations in healthcare PPE are starting to be seen in the marketplace, but much more needs to be done to move the design of PPE from an industrial perspective toward the realities of the healthcare workplace.

This chapter focuses on research on designing and engineering effective PPE. The chapter begins with a brief overview of the 2008 report, followed by a synopsis of research that has been conducted in the past several years. The chapter concludes with the committee's thoughts on research gaps and immediate and long-term research directions.

BACKGROUND AND CONTEXT
FROM THE 2008 REPORT

The 2008 Institute of Medicine (IOM) report provided the outline for a lifecycle approach to PPE and emphasized that, in addition to fit and filtration for respirators and functionality requirements for other types of PPE, numerous other factors play a significant role in the design and development of healthcare PPE. These factors include issues involving visibility, comfort and wearability, durability, maintenance and reuse, aesthetics, and cost (Figure 3-1).

In considering a framework for the design and development of PPE, the 2008 committee addressed the three phases of the design and engineering process typically associated with a product's lifecycle:

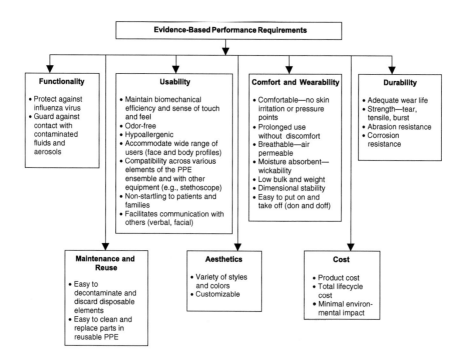

FIGURE 3-1 A structured approach to evidence-based performance requirements for personal protective equipment (PPE).
SOURCE: IOM (2008).

1. **User requirements analysis:** understanding the work hazards and barriers to PPE use;
2. **Design realization:** identifying the key characteristics (Figure 3-1) and translating the evidence-based performance requirements into the specific design of the PPE component while making appropriate trade-offs among the factors that drive design, including degree of protection, comfort, and the cost of designing the specific PPE component to meet the regulatory requirements; and
3. **Field use and evaluation:** requiring that the new PPE be tested in the field in order to provide a realistic assessment of its performance and to identify unintended consequences of use.

Fit and filtration are the major functional issues in the design and engineering of respirators. Most research has focused on filtration. National Institute for Occupational Safety and Health (NIOSH) ratings for respirators of 95, 99, or 100 percent filtration efficiency are based on the percentage of 0.3 μm particles that do not penetrate the test filter (IOM, 2008). Influenza viruses, with estimated sizes ranging from approximately 0.08 to 0.12 μm (although droplets with the virus can vary widely in size), follow standard particle filtration theory, and therefore a number of types of filters are effective. Less is known about issues regarding inward face seal leakage and other aspects of respirator fit. The 2008 report recommended research on a number of respirator issues, including decontamination and reuse methods, comfort and tolerability concerns, powered air-purifying respirators (PAPRs) designed to meet the needs of healthcare personnel, and improved face seals.

The 2008 report also addressed research for gowns, gloves, eye protection, face protection, and other types of PPE that might be needed to protect workers from infectious disease. These types of barrier protection are designed primarily to protect against droplet spray and contact transmission that might occur when particles are transferred to the respiratory mucosa or conjunctiva (of the eyes) of susceptible individuals within close range. Testing of gowns has focused primarily on liquid barrier performance and breathability of the fabric, with four levels of liquid barrier performance defined by the Association for the Advancement of Medical Instrumentation's (AAMI's) testing standard, AAMI PB70. The prior report emphasized the need to explore whether specific clinical situations require varying types of gowns or whether other specifications are needed, as well as issues regarding feasibility of reuse, interface with other types of PPE (especially gloves), and advances in materials technology, including repellant finishes (IOM, 2008). For protective eyewear, including transparent face shields, issues regarding the interface with respirators were found to be a critical need. In addition, product performance standards for eye protection need to be defined more clearly because they now focus on the thickness and impact resistance of eye protection but do not address issues relevant to influenza transmission (IOM, 2008).

Healthcare personnel's use of gloves can serve several purposes in infection control—creating a barrier to direct contact with contaminated surfaces, preventing patient-to-patient contamination if gloves are changed between patients and proper hand hygiene is performed, and increasing awareness of the potential for self-inoculation when gloved hands touch the mucosa of the mouth, nose, or eyes. Research needs regarding gloves that were identified in the 2008 report included better barrier protection as well as wearability and improved interfaces with gowns and other PPE. Adherence to hand hygiene and other infection control practices are also important in preventing disease transmission.

The 2008 report provided a list of immediate opportunities and long-term research needs for improving the design and effectiveness of healthcare PPE. The report also provided a set of recommendations in this area, which can be briefly summarized as follows:

- Define evidence-based performance requirements for PPE.
- Adopt a systems approach to the design and development of PPE.
- Increase research on the design and engineering of the next generation of PPE.
- Establish measures to assess and compare the effectiveness of PPE.

UPDATE ON RECENT RESEARCH

Research efforts since the prior report have continued to address a range of design and engineering issues with the goal of improving the PPE available to healthcare personnel and others. The following section provides an overview of recent research efforts, beginning with the research focused on respirators and face masks.

Respirators and Face Masks: Fit and Filtration

The protection provided by a particular respirator is a function of both the filtration capabilities of the material and how well the device fits the wearer. Total inward leakage (TIL) is the combination of filtration, face seal leakage, and leakage through respirator components, such as the exhalation valve.

Filtration

Several issues concerning filtration have been raised recently. First, the filtration efficiency of face masks is a concern because they are not developed as filtration devices. Second, researchers have been concerned about the penetration of nanoparticles (which includes the size range of influenza and other viruses) through respirator filter media and whether current NIOSH respirator certification methods accurately account for those particles. Third, shortages of respiratory protection may occur during a pandemic, so alternative filter materials and equipment have been investigated.

Filtration efficiency of face masks Two recent studies investigated the filtration efficiency of face masks. Oberg and Brosseau (2008) evaluated filtration performance of nine face masks (cup, flat, duckbill, one and two straps, ear loops, surgical, laser, and procedure). Filter efficiencies ranged from 0 to 84 percent for the latex sphere tests and 4 to 90 percent in the sodium chloride (NaCl) tests. Dental masks showed significantly higher penetration (6 to 75 percent for latex and 53 to 90 percent for salt) than hospital masks (0.02 to 0.7 percent for latex and 4 to 37 percent for salt). Only 1 of the hospital masks (mask H) had less than 5 percent penetration of the salt particles. Lee and colleagues (2008c) investigated the protection factor of face masks and respirators with a challenge of particles representing bacterial and viral size ranges (aerodynamic size: 0.04 to 1.3 μm) and found that none of the masks had protection factors > 10. The protection factors of the tested N95 respirators were an average of 8 to 12 times greater than those of masks. One previous study (Li et al., 2006) reported that face masks provided 95 percent filtration efficiency for potassium chloride. However, Brosseau and Harriman (2007) pointed out that the study did not use a standard method and that the authors did not fully describe the technique. None of the face masks tested by Oberg and Brosseau (2008) or Lee and colleagues (2008c) provided sufficient protection to be considered respirators. This is not surprising considering the fact that face masks were not intended to be respiratory protective equipment.

Penetration of small particles NIOSH certification tests for N95 respirators use an NaCl aerosol challenge with a 300 nm most penetrating particle size (MPPS).[1] However, many electret filter media that use electrostatic charge to capture particles have an MPPS ranging from 30 to 100 nm (Shaffer and Rengasamy, 2009). Concerns have been raised regarding the filtration performance of N95 respirators against smaller viral- and bacterial-sized particles. Eninger and colleagues (2008b) reviewed the NIOSH aerosol particle-size distribution and measurement method. The authors found that, although the salt aerosol does contain a significant fraction of ultrafine (diameters < 100 nm) particles, the method and equipment used cannot accurately measure the contributions of particles below 100 nm. In fact, 68 percent by count and 8 percent by mass of salt particles below 100 nm did not significantly contribute to the filter penetration measurement. Therefore, the existing NIOSH certification protocol may not adequately reflect the penetration of ultrafine particles.

Several groups of researchers have investigated the filtration performance of respirators against nanoparticles. Eninger and colleagues (2008a) investigated the filtration performance of one N95 and two N99 filtering facepiece respirators against one inert particle and three virus aerosols at flow rates of 30, 85, and 150 L/min. The respirators were sealed on a manikin. The most penetrating particle size for challenge aerosols was < 0.1 μm for all three respirators. Mean particle penetration, by count, was increased significantly when the size fraction of particles < 0.1 μm was included compared to particles > 0.1 μm. Penetration of the salt aerosol was greater than that of the tested biological aerosols, suggesting that inert aerosols can be used to assess filter penetration of virions. Inhalation airflow rate had a significant effect on particle penetration. The authors suggested that further research is needed with cyclic flows with high peak inspiratory flows.

A study of the filtration performance of five N95 and two P100 filtering facepiece respirators against monodisperse silver aerosol particles

---

[1]The MPPS is the particle size that has the lowest filtration efficiency. Particles near the MPPS are too large to be efficiently captured by diffusion, but they are too small to be efficiently captured by the filtration mechanisms of impaction and interception.

in the 4 to 30 nm range at 85 L/min found that both types of respirators showed a decrease in percentage of penetration, with a decrease in particle diameter down to 4 nm (Rengasamy et al., 2008). This study supports prior studies that indicate that NIOSH-approved air-purifying respirators provided expected filtration protection against nanoparticles. A follow-up study using a polydisperse NaCl aerosol test with a 238 nm mass median aerodynamic diameter and two monodisperse aerosol tests concluded that the eight filtering facepiece respirator models tested met expected filtration performance against nanoparticles (Rengasamy et al., 2009). The NIOSH-certified respirators have a minimum efficiency of 95 percent for the N95 and 99.97 percent for the P100. The European Norm requires a minimum efficiency of 94 percent for a filtering facepiece respirator class P2 (FFP2) and 99 percent for a filtering facepiece respirator class P3 (FFP3). Penetrations from the polydisperse aerosol test were < 1 percent for the N95 and FFP2 models and < 0.03 percent for the P100 and FFP3 models.

In a study by Eshbaugh and colleagues (2009), the researchers examined the effects of varying flow conditions on aerosol penetration for both N95 and P100 filtering facepiece respirators and cartridges. Challenges were inert solids and oil aerosols with particle sizes in the range of 0.02 to 2.9 μm; three constant flow and four cyclic flow conditions were used. Penetration increased under increasing constant- and cyclic-flow conditions. The MPPS for the P100 filters was 50 to 200 nm and 50 nm for N95 filters. Shaffer and Rengasamy (2009) reviewed research published since 2000 on respirator filtration and leakage data for nanoparticles. The MPPS was in the 30 to 100 nm range and was impacted by the filter media and test conditions, particularly flow rate. They found that filtration of monodisperse nanoparticles at the MPPS varied from 1.4 to 10 percent for the N95 filtering facepiece respirator. They identified the greatest need for further research as human laboratory or workplace protection factor studies to measure TIL for respirators used for protection against nanoparticles. Wander and Heimbuch (2009) tested one N95 and one P100 filtering facepiece respirator with aerosolized particles (count mode diameter ~0.8 μm) of H1N1 and inert beads at 85 L/min using the Laboratory-Scale Aerosol Tunnel. The N95 removed > 99 percent of viable H1N1 while the P100 removed > 99.99 percent. They performed the same against the inert beads. The authors concluded that infectious microorganisms and inert particles of the same size have the same impact on the filtering efficiency of filtering facepiece respirators.

Although these studies used different challenge aerosols and different test methods, several common results emerge. Inhalation airflow rate had a significant effect on particle penetration (Eninger et al., 2008a; Eshbaugh et al., 2009). NIOSH- or European Norm–certified filtering facepiece respirators achieved expected filtration performance when challenged with nanoparticle aerosols (Eninger et al., 2008a; Eshbaugh et al., 2009; Rengasamy et al., 2008, 2009). The MPPS is below 100 nm for most electret filter media (Eninger et al., 2008a; Eshbaugh et al., 2009; Rengasamy et al., 2009), though one researcher (Eshbaugh et al., 2009) reported 200 nm for two models of filtering facepiece respirators. Finally, inert particles have penetration performance similar to virus particles (Eninger et al., 2008a; Wander and Heimbuch, 2009).

Alternative filter materials In the event of a pandemic, there may not be enough respirators available to meet demand. Rengasamy and colleagues (2010a) examined the filtration performance of common cloth materials, such as sweatshirts, T-shirts, towels, scarves, and cloth masks, against nanoparticles using polydisperse and monodisperse aerosols (20 to 1,000 nm) at two face velocities. The cloth materials had penetration levels of 40 to 90 percent for polydispersed NaCl, well above that of N95 respirators. Penetrations of 9 to 98 percent were obtained for different monodisperse NaCl aerosol nanoparticles. These materials had penetration levels similar to some face masks that were tested previously. They concluded that only minimal protection would be provided by wearing masks made out of these cloth materials, especially when considering that face seal leakage will decrease protection further.

Fit

Face seal leakage is a critical factor in the amount of protection provided by a respirator. Although much research has been done on filtering media and improving filter efficiency, the fit side of the equation has not been explored in such depth. Several recent studies examined aspects of fit related to healthcare personnel.

Face masks Two recent studies examined the extent to which face masks fit the face. Duling and colleagues (2007) assessed six face masks. The simulated workplace protection factor fifth percentile value was 1.4 and the lower 90 percent confidence limit was 1.2, indicating that none of the masks provided adequate protection. Oberg and Brosseau (2008) evaluated facial fit of 5 face masks using qualitative and quantitative fit tests with 20 human volunteers. When the subjects put on the face masks themselves, they all failed the qualitative fit test. When they were assisted with donning the face masks, 18 subjects failed the fit test. For unassisted donning, average quantitative fit factors were 2.5 to 6.9; for assisted donning, they ranged from 2.8 to 9.6. None of the masks tested attained an individual fit factor of 100, the minimum passing level required by the Occupational Safety and Health Administration (OSHA) for a half-mask filtering facepiece respirator.

Loose-fitting PAPRs Loose-fitting PAPRs may be worn by healthcare personnel who have beards or who cannot otherwise wear an N95 filtering-facepiece or elastomeric air-purifying respirator. The unfiltered, exhaled air from the PAPR may transmit virus from the wearer to others. An N95 respirator may be worn inside the PAPR to prevent this from happening. Roberge and colleagues (2008) used a manikin to assess the protection factor of a loose-fitting PAPR with and without an N95 respirator glued to the manikin. Flow rates were 25 L/min and 40 L/min. The N95 significantly increased the PAPR protection factor even when the PAPR blower was turned off. However, consideration should be given to the possible negative impact of the additional physiological burden of wearing an N95 respirator inside a PAPR (Roberge, 2008). Additionally, their results might not hold in the work setting because the N95 was glued to the face (Roberge et al., 2008). Some loose-fitting PAPRs do not fully encapsulate the head, making it possible for the wearer to overbreathe the blower and possibly be exposed to contaminants (Roberge et al., 2008). Johnson and colleagues (2008) found that the 1.1 L of air inside the loose-fitting PAPR they tested would act as a buffer against contaminated air that leaks into the respirator due to overbreathing the blower. That volume could also help if an N95 were worn under the PAPR and face seal leaks occurred.

Fit testing and inward leakage Several large-scale fit tests of healthcare personnel were completed recently (Lee et al., 2008b; McMahon et al., 2008; Oestenstad et al., 2007; Wilkinson et al., 2010; Winter et al., 2010). McMahon and colleagues (2008) found that 5 percent of men and 15 percent of women could not pass the fit test with the first respirator tried, while Lee and colleagues (2008b) had 26 percent of workers fail the fit test with the first respirator. Winter and colleagues (2010) found that 28 percent of 50 staff members did not fit the 3 respirators tested. Wilkinson and colleagues (2010) found that 82.9 percent of 6,160 healthcare personnel were successfully fitted with the first respirator, 12.3 percent required testing with a second respirator, and 4.8 percent required testing with 3 or more respirators. Therefore, multiple respirators are likely to be needed to get passing fit tests for all staff. First-time pass rates may improve after NIOSH incorporates the new sizing panels (Zhuang et al., 2007, 2008) into its TIL certification requirement.

Gender and age in women may be significant factors in achieving a successful fit (McMahon et al., 2008), though Oestenstad and colleagues (2007) did not find a gender difference in the 41 subjects they tested. Gender, respirator brand, and test repetition did not have any significant effects on location or shape of leaks assessed on half-mask respirators using a fluorescent tracer during fit tests (Oestenstad and Bartolucci, 2010). There was a difference in fit test leak-site distribution for women, and the authors suggested that facial dimensions may be an important factor. In fact, their prior research showed that fit was significantly associated with face length and lip width and possibly face width (Oestenstad et al., 2007). Weight gain during pregnancy may impact fit due to changes in facial anthropometrics (Roberge, 2009). Wilkinson and colleagues (2010) found that personnel who reported their race as Asian had the highest failure rate and that race was correlated with facial shape. Training improved the fit test pass rate (Lee et al., 2008b; Winter et al., 2010). However, as time elapsed from the fit test, pass rates were similar to those prior to training, although frequent use after training led to increased pass rates (Lee et al., 2008b).

Experience of the fit testers was found to be a significant factor in achieving a successful fit test with the first respirator tried (Wilkinson et al., 2010). Their testers selected a respirator based on observations of the subject's facial characteristics, the physical fit of the respirator, and the "real-time" option on the PortaCount® fit tester. Janssen and colleagues (2007) evaluated the workplace protection factor of an N95 filtering facepiece respirator during light, moderate, and heavy intensity tasks in a steel foundry and found a large variability in protection because of removing and re-donning the respirator. This may also be a problem in healthcare settings. They suggested that a time-weighted, average workplace protection factor be considered to estimate ongoing protection.

Participants at a NIOSH-sponsored workshop (Brosseau, 2009) expressed interest in developing a respirator that did not require initial and annual fit tests and provided suggestions for improving the fit capabilities of respirators. Au and colleagues (2010) proposed using a customizable, reusable mask with high-efficiency air filters. They investigated the efficacy of this mask without fit testing versus a fit tested N95 respirator in 22 volunteers. The median filtration factor was significantly higher for the N95 respirators compared to the mask that is cut to size. Only 16 of the 22 volunteers had a fit factor greater than 100. This was lower than the pass rate for the N95 (19/22), but was not significantly different. The authors concluded that the customizable mask should be studied further, but that it should not be used without fit testing at this time.

Face seal leakage is an important factor in respirator protection, and it depends on several factors, including proper respirator selection, fit, and donning. Cho and colleagues (2010) found that most particle penetration occurs through face seal leakage even when the respirator fits well (workplace protection factor = 515), and that particle penetration of the face seal decreases with increases in breathing rate and particle size. Similarly, Grinshpun and colleagues (2009) found that the number of particles penetrating through the facepiece seal far exceeded penetration through the filter medium for both an N95 respirator and a face mask using challenge particles in the 0.03 to 1 μm range. Lee and colleagues (2008c) investigated the protection factor of four N95 respirators and three face masks with a challenge of particles representing bacterial and viral size ranges (aerodynamic size: 0.04 to 1.3 μm). Prior research (Coffey et al., 2004) had demonstrated high protection levels for Respirator A and medium protection for Respirator B. Respirators C and D were the same except D had an exhalation valve. Overall, 29 percent of N95 respirators and 100 percent of face masks had protection factors of < 10, the assigned protection factor for the N95 (Lee et al., 2008c). The percentages of N95 respirators with protection factors of > 10 for all particle sizes tested were 86, 36, 89, and 78 percent for Respirators A to D, respectively. There were no significant differences in the protection factor between the N95 and N95 with the exhalation valve. The protection factors of the N95 were an average of 8 to 12 times greater than those of face masks.

Particle size–dependent face seal leakage has not been fully investigated (Shaffer and Rengasamy, 2009). However, NIOSH has initiated studies to determine whether face seal leakage of nanoparticles is consistent with the leakages observed for gases/vapors and larger particles. Further research on leakage of nanoparticles is important to better understand the effectiveness of filtering facepiece respirators in workplaces where nanoparticles are present.

Preventing a Patient from Spreading Virus

One suggestion for protecting personnel from virus exposure is to place a face mask or N95 respirator on a patient with confirmed influenza. Huang and Huang (2007) demonstrated greater bacterial leakage at close range for a face mask (15.8 percent of no mask control) than for an N95 respirator (4.1 percent of control). Placing positively charged polypropylene edging on the mask and respirator decreased leakage to 4.5 and 1.8 percent of control, respectively. This indicates that masks and respirators could be modified easily to decrease virus transfer.

Tang and colleagues (2009) used a schlieren optical method to visualize cough flows of volunteers wearing either a face mask or N95 respirator. With the N95, more of the cough went through the front of the respirator compared to the face mask, and the N95 was better at preventing leakage of the cough. The face mask on the standing people who coughed blocked the forward motion of the cough jet and directed it upward, downward, and out of the sides of the mask. The leakage air from both the mask and respirator had little momentum. They concluded that both face masks and N95 respirators decelerated and redirected the expelled air, which then joined the general upward motion of the cougher's thermal plume created by body heat. This prevented the cough from being projected forward as a rapid turbulent jet over distances sufficient to reach the breathing zones of other individuals.

Diaz and Smaldone (2010) recently developed a headform-based system to evaluate the effectiveness of N95 respirators and loose- or tight-fitting face masks in preventing transmission of infectious aerosols from a source to a receiver. Although an N95 on the source filtered significantly more particles than the face masks, the simulated workplace protection factor did not differ for the unmasked receiver. When the receiver wore each mask or respirator, < 1 percent of the particles were filtered and the simulated workplace protection factor was 1.4 to 2.2. Sealing an N95 to the source using Vaseline® yielded a simulated workplace protection factor of 4,082, and sealing it to the receiver resulted in a protection factor of 118. The authors concluded that the face masks worn at the source resulted in greater protection than a face mask or respirator worn on the receiver.

Both Huang and Huang (2007) and Tang and colleagues (2009) showed greater leakage with the face mask than with the N95 respirator. This seems to contrast with the results of Johnson and colleagues (2009), who showed that both fully blocked virus expulsion. However, Huang and Huang as well as Tang and colleagues considered leakage from the sides of the face mask and respirator, while Johnson and colleagues had volunteers cough directly onto the collection plate. Although Tang and colleagues (2009) indicated that the cough flow was directed away from the receiver, they did not assess filtration, so virus particles that could not be observed with the schlieren optics could have reached the receiver. Diaz and Smaldone (2010) did not use heated manikins, so there were no thermal plumes that may have directed the particle flow upward and away from the receiver. More research is needed to understand the particle dynamics of exhaled viruses while wearing a face mask or respirator in order to make a recommendation regarding patient mask or respirator wear.

Summary: Respirator and Face Masks—Fit and Filtration

Several studies have shown that face masks do not have sufficient filtration or fit to provide adequate inhalation protection of small particles to wearers. NIOSH-certified N95 respirators have been shown by several studies to provide expected filtration levels of nanoparticles. However, high filtration efficiency alone does not ensure that the wearer will be protected. Mask D in Oberg and Brosseau's study (2008) had the second highest filtration efficiency, but the lowest fit factor. Because face seal leakage far exceeds penetration through the filter (Cho et al., 2010; Grinshpun et al., 2009), future research should focus on improving respirator fit.

Although Lee and colleagues (2008c) showed that some N95 respirators may not achieve an assigned protection factor of 10 when nanoparticles are present, whether higher fit factors would have been achieved with a different model respirator is unknown. The rates of failure from their study were similar to the fit-factor failure rates of large-scale protection-factor tests performed on healthcare personnel (Lee et al., 2008b; McMahon et al., 2008; Winter et al., 2010). Multiple respirators should be available for healthcare personnel, as currently required by OSHA's respirator standard, because it is unlikely that one model or size will fit all employees. Long-term storage of these additional respirators should have little impact on penetration levels (Viscusi et al., 2009a). Participants in a no-fit respirator workshop (Brosseau, 2009) identified the need for a user seal check that works, continuous fit checking rather than a no-fit test, and a respirator that can be put on easily multiple times.

These features would be beneficial because protection varies with repeated donning (Janssen et al., 2007).

Respirators: Decontamination

Reuse of filtering facepiece respirators has been suggested as a strategy to counteract anticipated supply shortages during a pandemic and to reduce costs. The potential for the respirator to serve as a fomite is a serious concern. Safe, effective decontamination methods that inactivate the virus without altering the respirator performance and physical characteristics are necessary for this to occur. Respirators impregnated with antiviral particles may decrease the risk of virus transmission because of improper handling of virus-exposed protective equipment. To study this issue, methods are first needed to effectively deposit virus onto respirators, and then their potential to act as fomites can be investigated. Finally, the effectiveness of treated filter media and decontamination methods can be assessed.

To assess the efficacy of decontamination methods, reliable and repeatable methods of applying contaminant aerosols to filter media are needed. NIOSH has developed two systems for applying virus aerosols to respirator filter media that pass the aerosol through the filter media rather than depositing it on the surface. The bioaerosol respirator test system (Fisher et al., 2009) loads filter media with virus-containing particles while the droplet-phase aerosol respirator test system (Vo et al., 2009) applies droplets onto media. Another system, the Dry Aerosol Deposition Device (Heimbuch et al., 2009), deposits biological aerosols onto the surface using impaction, a system that allows the aerosol to be delivered quickly and with reproducible loading.

Additionally, to assess the number of viable particles on PPE, recovery methods are needed that allow removal without killing the virus. Casanova and colleagues (2009) developed a new technique for recovering bacteriophage MS2, a non-enveloped virus, from contaminated gloves, gowns, respirators, and goggles. Recovered viruses were not inactivated, indicating that this technique can be used for viral survival studies.

Rate and length of virus survival are key facts needed to assess the potential for respirators to serve as fomites. Rengasamy and colleagues (2010b) applied MS2 as both an aerosol and as liquid drops onto N95 filter coupons. They demonstrated that > 10 percent of the challenge

MS2 bacteriophage survived for 20 hours at 22°C and 30 percent relative humidity. Fisher and Shaffer (2010) subsequently assessed MS2 survivability at 1, 2, 3, 4, 5, and 10 days. The authors found that 10 percent of initial MS2 survived for 4 days for both deposition methods, and that all samples had detectable levels of MS2 on the tenth day. Because MS2 is a non-enveloped virus, enveloped influenza virus survivability cannot be estimated from the current study. MS2 survives for longer periods of time on surfaces than influenza does. Because fomites may be a source for indirect contact transmission, decontamination may be required before reuse.

Decontamination Methods

Studies of various types of decontamination methods have not yet been successful in identifying an effective means for decontamination that does not affect the structure and integrity of the respirator. Viscusi and coworkers (2007, 2009b) assessed the effect of decontamination methods on filter aerosol penetration, physical appearance, and airflow resistance. From their initial list of 10 potential decontamination methods (autoclave, isopropyl alcohol, bleach, hydrogen peroxide, microwave, soap and water, ultraviolet [UV] radiation, dry heat, vaporized hydrogen peroxide, and ethylene oxide) (2007), liquid hydrogen peroxide, vaporized hydrogen peroxide, and UV radiation caused the least change in filter performance. The authors (2009b) then further evaluated five decontamination methods (UV germicidal irradiation, ethylene oxide, vaporized hydrogen peroxide, microwave oven irradiation, and bleach) on three models each of N95, P100, and surgical N95 filtering facepiece respirators. Ethylene oxide and UV germicidal irradiation were the only methods that did not cause any observable physical changes to the respirators. The bleach method left a noticeable odor, even after overnight drying, and bleach off-gassed when the decontaminated respirators were rehydrated with deionized water. UV germicidal irradiation, ethylene oxide, and vaporized hydrogen peroxide were the most promising decontamination methods, although there are concerns regarding throughput for the latter two methods.

Fisher and colleagues (2009) investigated a process for applying viral droplets to respirators to evaluate decontamination methods. Two decontamination methods, one physical (steam) and one chemical (bleach), were examined as well as two concentrations of organic matter (protective factor) in the aerosol medium. The organic matter had a protein concentration similar to the organic challenge in ASTM E1053-97, *Standard Test Method for Efficacy of Virucidal Agents Intended for Inanimate Environmental Surfaces*. The organic matter may protect the virus by neutralizing the decontamination solution or by providing a physical barrier to the decontaminant. Detectable differences were noted in the efficacy of the bleach decontamination, depending on the concentration of bleach and protective factor. Steam showed an effect for treatment time, but not protective factor. Viruses recovered were more likely to be found on the outer layer than when low concentrations of organic matter were used. This would be important for a decontamination method such as UV light that only reaches the outer layer of filter material.

A study of bleach and UV radiation (Vo et al., 2009) found that bleach concentration and UV exposure time were factors in decontamination. UV radiation was recommended for further study, such as assessing the impact of pleats or folds in filtering facepiece respirators, because it was non-toxic and did not leave an odor. Low-dose UV radiation resulted in 3-$\log_{10}$ reductions in MS2, while higher doses resulted in no detectable MS2. The authors discussed that further research is needed because non-enveloped MS2 may not behave in the same manner as enveloped viruses, and because the composition and size of particles used might not exactly mimic respiratory secretions.

Finally, Salter and colleagues (2010) assessed the amount of residual chemicals on six models of filtering facepiece respirators after seven decontamination methods: ethylene oxide, vaporized hydrogen peroxide, UV light, and four liquids (hydrogen peroxide, bleach, mixed oxidants, and dimethyl dioxirane). Six of the seven methods did not deposit significant amounts of toxic residue. The ethylene oxide–treated respirators had detectable levels of 2-hydroxyethyl acetate, a hazardous byproduct that may have been formed when the ethylene oxide reacted with rubber parts of the respirator. As noted by other authors, bleach-treated respirators had a bleach odor after treatment. The bleach also corroded metal parts and discolored others. Dimethyl dioxirane and mixed oxidants also oxidized metal parts and had distinct odors.

Practical decontamination methods are needed as decontamination of filtering facepiece respirators is not currently an option. Although bleach is readily available and inexpensive, it has been shown to cause offensive odors and can cause corrosion. Ethylene oxide may react with rubber straps to create a hazardous byproduct. It also has problems with throughput, as does vaporized hydrogen peroxide. Other techniques such as soap and water, isopropyl alcohol, and microwaving can cause changes to the physical characteristics of the respirator. UV radiation shows promise, although its effectiveness on inner filter layers and pleats is unknown, as is its affect on electrostatic properties of electret filters. Additional research with enveloped influenza viruses is needed.

Treated Filter Media

Several studies investigated the decontamination efficacy of treated filter media. Oxford and colleagues (2007) found that masks impregnated with QR-435, a green tea extract mix, trapped a significantly greater amount of virus compared to an untreated mask. Lee and colleagues (2008a) exposed iodine-treated filter media to aerosolized bacteria at an equivalent of 85 L/min flow. Viability of collected spores from control and treated media were assessed. Survival fraction was significantly lower for the treated filter versus untreated at room temperature and low relative humidity. However, there were no differences in viability at room temperature and high relative humidity or at high temperature and high relative humidity. Lee and colleagues (2009) then investigated the efficacy of iodine-treated filter media against MS2 aerosols. Treated media showed significantly higher viable removal efficiencies than untreated. Rengasamy and colleagues (2010b) applied MS2 virus droplet nuclei onto four coupons from antimicrobial respirators and controls. Antimicrobial agents included iodine, embedded silver-copper throughout the fibers of the outer layer of the mask, EnvizO3-Shield technology on the outer layer, and titanium dioxide–coated filter layers beneath the outer layer. MS2 is less sensitive to many antimicrobial agents because it is a non-enveloped virus, which is hardier and able to survive longer than enveloped viruses such as influenza. The iodinated fibers from Respirator C had a significant increase in the $\log_{10}$ reduction of MS2 at 37°C and 80 percent relative humidity, but not at lower temperatures and relative humidity. MS2 droplet nuclei survived for more than 20 hours at room temperature and 30 percent relative humidity. For an antimicrobial agent to be effective, it needs to reduce viability faster. At 22°C, 30 percent relative humidity, all four antimicrobial respirators had $< 1 \log_{10}$ reduction, which was not significantly different from the control. The iodinated respirator showed 3.7 $\log_{10}$ reduction of MS2 at 4 hours. This was significantly higher than the control, while the others were not significantly different from the control. Therefore, the decontamination efficacy of the antimicrobial respirators depends on storage conditions and the antimicrobial agent. Iodine from the filter that enters the extraction medium may also inactivate virus.

Borkow and colleagues (2010) investigated the antiviral properties of a copper oxide–containing N95 respirator. Treated and control respirators were exposed to aerosolized human influenza A virus and avian influenza virus at a constant airflow rate for 1 minute. The number of infectious virus titers recovered from the masks was measured 30 minutes after exposure. The researchers found that the copper oxide particles did not impact filtration efficiency, but there was a statistically significant difference in retrieved infectious influenza between the control and copper oxide–impregnated masks. This could offer the possibility of reducing the risk of hand or environmental contamination, with potential subsequent infection due to improper handling of exposed respirators.

Summary: Decontamination

Various techniques have been developed for applying viruses to respirators. Recent research has shown that non-enveloped viruses can persist on respirators for up to 10 days in hospital-like environments (Fisher and Shaffer, 2010). Although enveloped viruses such as the influenza virus may not survive as long, it is reasonable to assume that the virus will survive long enough to render the respirator a potential fomite. Current decontamination research has not demonstrated an effective technique for killing viruses that does not also have a detrimental impact on respirator physical characteristics or function. More research in this area is needed. Iodine-treated and copper oxide–impregnated filter media show promise for inactivating virus in the respirator.

Respirators: Tolerance, Physiological Responses, and Communications

Respirators worn by healthcare personnel have the potential to impact comfort, physiological responses, task performance, and communications with each other and with patients. Protective equipment, such as respirators or face shields, may create pressure points that cause discomfort. The breathing resistance and dead volume of the respirators may alter respiration and lead to a build-up of carbon dioxide. Because respirators may alter the wearer's field of view, some tasks may be more difficult to perform and thus may take longer. The respirator covers the mouth, muffling speech and removing visual cues for the listener. Additionally, the noise created by a PAPR blower and environmental noise both hinder communications. Several researchers have investigated the impact of respirators on healthcare personnel.

Respirator Tolerance

Consistent use of PPE by healthcare personnel during exposure to hazards is essential to achieve the benefits afforded by the devices. One of the critical features in helping to achieve consistent compliance in the wearing of PPE may be the comfort and tolerability of the equipment itself.

Although most healthcare personnel appear to be assigned N95 respirators for use, elastomeric respirators represent an alternative type of respiratory protection that could be used. Roberge and colleagues (2010c) reported the comfort responses of healthcare personnel wearing a half-face elastomeric respirator who completed exercise regimes for a 1-hour period. The healthcare personnel's mean comfort scores were low, indicating that the elastomeric respirators were generally comfortable, and the comfort scores were not significantly different from controls (no respirator). Complaints of subjective symptoms and design features of the respirator included facial heat, skin irritation, and weight of the respirator, among others.

Little is known about the tolerability of healthcare personnel to wearing respirators, particularly during an influenza pandemic where they likely would be required to be worn for long periods of time within an 8-hour work shift over a duration involving a number of weeks or more. Radonovich and colleagues (2009) determined the mean tolerance time that healthcare personnel would be willing to wear a variety of respirator ensembles (including N95s, PAPRs, half-face elastomerics, and face masks in various combinations) while performing their normal job duties. Healthcare personnel stopped wearing their respirator ensemble before the end of an 8-hour shift in 59 percent of the total work shifts evaluated by the study. Reasons given for discontinued wear included communication difficulties (visual, auditory, or vocal), heat, pressure or pain, and dizziness or difficulty concentrating, among others. Median tolerance times varied by the respirator ensemble worn, ranging from 4.1

to 7.7 hours. Wearers of disposable models often complained of facial heat and pressure, while users of reusable models often reported communication problems. A cup-shaped N95 with an exhalation valve had a greater median tolerance time (7.7 hours) compared to a similar model that was not equipped with a valve (5.8 hours). The ensemble combination of cup N95 plus a face mask had the shortest median tolerance time of 4.1 hours. The PAPR had a slightly lower median tolerance time (7.6 hours) than either the cup-shaped N95 with exhalation valve or face mask, which had the same median tolerance time (7.7 hours). Although the difference is not likely to be clinically significant, it is surprising that the tolerance time for the PAPR was lower than that for the N95 with exhalation valve. It is also interesting to note that the tolerance time for the face mask was similar to both the PAPR and the N95 with exhalation valve. However, the N95 with exhalation valve had a higher number of complaints (24) than the PAPR (17) or face mask (17).

Harber and colleagues (2009) evaluated a number of subjective tolerance measures to respirator use by subjects selected from the general population, including some with mild respiratory impairment, while engaging in exercise and work simulation. Respirators evaluated included half-face elastomerics and N95s. Under work simulation, the subjective tolerance measures (e.g., comfort, heat, speech) for all variables assessed, except heat, were more "adverse" for the elastomeric half-mask respirator than for the N95. The largest adverse subjective ratings were for comfort, face, breathing, heat, and heavy weight of the device. The largest differences between the two types of respirators were for subjective measures of nose impact and heavy weight, with the elastomeric model demonstrating the greater adverse impact among subjects on these two measures. Overall, however, the study concluded that while both respirator types were "relatively well tolerated," N95 respirators may be preferable to elastomeric respirators.

Although not much is known about what workers would like to see incorporated into future respirator designs to assist in increasing compliance, one recent study surveyed healthcare personnel to assess their perspectives on this issue (Baig et al., 2010). Of 149 survey respondents, only 24 percent reported that their N95 respirator was comfortable most of the time or always, and only 6 percent indicated that they would be able to tolerate wearing an N95 respirator continuously for an 8-hour shift. Overall, 56 percent of respondents believe there is a need to develop a new N95 respirator for healthcare personnel, 44 percent preferred an N95 that does not require fit testing, and 60 percent preferred wearing a disposable device. Problems identified by respondents that need to be addressed in future respirator design included discomfort, difficulty breathing, heat, and low tolerability for use over extended time periods.

Physiological Impact

The physiological impact of respirators on workers is an important factor in designing wearable PPE. Recent studies have investigated the physiological impact of respirators during physical tasks and while walking on a treadmill. Vojtko and colleagues (2008) found small but statistically significant increases in both inhalation and exhalation resistances of a face mask placed over an N95 filtering facepiece respirator for minute volumes of 25 and 40 L/min, but the total did not exceed NIOSH limits (although those are measured at 85 L/min). Although their study was performed with a simulator, the authors concluded that the slight increases in resistance should not impact the wearer's respiratory effort.

Bansal and colleagues (2009) assessed the impact of one dual-cartridge elastomeric and one N95 half-face mask respirator on both normal and respiratory-impaired volunteers (respiratory impairments were listed as chronic rhinitis, mild chronic obstructive pulmonary disease, and mild asthma). No control condition was used. Sedentary (bolt sorting), low-intensity (walk across room and put papers in appropriate bins), and moderate-intensity (stock shelves with cereal boxes and juice jugs) tasks were included. The authors found small but statistically significant differences between the two respirators for inhalation time (longer for half-face models, 1.14 versus 1.10), exhalation time (shorter for half-face models, 1.39 versus 1.44), and increased duty cycle for half-face models (0.46 versus 0.45). However, the differences are not likely to be clinically significant. The authors stated that neither respirator should cause hypoventilation and that both types of respirators should be well tolerated for most individuals, including those with mild respiratory impairments.

Another study used thermal imaging to assess surface temperature of two N95 respirators and two N95 respirators with exhalation valves from the same manufacturer (Monaghan et al., 2009). Respirators were placed on a headform with an Automated Breathing Metabolic Simulator supplying air at 100 percent relative humidity and 33°C at 10 L/min for an hour. The authors concluded that at the breathing rate used, exhalation valves provided no heat dissipation benefits over a mask without one.

However, they also noted that the exhalation valve was not activated at the low breathing rate.

Roberge and colleagues (2010a,b,c) completed a number of studies that assessed the physiological impact of various respirators during a 1-hour treadmill walk at 1.7 and 2.5 mph. There were no significant differences between N95 filtering facepiece respirators with and without exhalation valves and the control in physiological variables, exertion scores, or comfort scores. The comparison of the N95 with and without the exhalation valve found no differences in the partial pressure of carbon dioxide (CO_2). Similar results were reported for face masks worn over the N95s either with or without the exhalation valve. The authors did note that face masks decreased oxygen levels in the filtering facepiece respirators at the low work rate and in the respirators with the exhalation valves at the higher work rate. An elastomeric air-purifying respirator resulted in decreased breathing rates and higher tidal volumes at both work rates, although the minute ventilation did not differ. While transcutaneous CO_2 values did not statistically differ (elastomeric air-purifying respirator versus control), some subjects had elevated levels that the authors suggested should be investigated further.

The elastomeric air-purifying respirator imposed little additional physiological burden over an hour of wear at the work rates assessed. Exhalation valves in N95 respirators may decrease exhalation resistance and help dissipate heat and CO_2 build-up; however, at low flow rates, these benefits may not be realized. Monaghan and coworkers (2009) noted that the exhalation valve was not activated at 10 L/min ventilation rate. This means wearers may not notice any difference in thermal sensation of the face during sedentary or low-intensity activities. Roberge and colleagues (2010b) found that at low work rates, excess CO_2 was not a problem. Therefore, the benefit of the exhalation valve may be seen only at higher work rates.

Healthy workers and those with mild respiratory impairments should be able to physiologically tolerate respirators. Little physiological burden should be imposed by filtering facepiece respirators (with or without a face mask) or by elastomeric respirators. However, the impact of filtering facepiece respirators on pregnant women is not well understood (Roberge, 2009). Respirators designed to accommodate the respiratory limitations of pregnant healthcare personnel may improve comfort and tolerability for other wearers (Roberge, 2009). Although loose-fitting PAPRs were not investigated, they should not impose a respiratory burden due to their positive air flow. However, the weight of the blower may increase the physiological workload.

Communications

Healthcare personnel must be able to communicate effectively and accurately with each other and with patients while wearing PPE. Communications while wearing PPE typical of healthcare personnel has been investigated by Mendel and colleagues (2008) and Radonovich and colleagues (2010). A third study involving air traffic controllers also provides useful information (Hah et al., 2009).

Mendel and coworkers (2008) assessed the impact of face masks on speech intelligibility using the Connected Speech Test with normal and hearing-impaired listeners in either a quiet room or with prerecorded noise from a dental drill played at 45 dBA. No impact was reported on speech intelligibility for either the normal or hearing-impaired listeners. A small but significant difference in scores for both mask and no-mask scores was noted due to background noise. Radonovich and coauthors (2010) used a Modified Rhyme Test with modified scoring to investigate the impact of face masks and respirators on speech communications. Reported scores were not corrected for guessing. The first set of trials was performed in an intensive care unit (ICU) room with simulated noise, with only the speaker wearing the device. The scores of the N95 cup-shaped respirator, duck bill N95, face mask, and control were statistically the same at both 3 and 7 feet in an ICU room with simulated noise. The elastomeric half-mask respirator with exhalation valve was the worst performer at 72 percent, scoring even lower than the loose-fitting PAPR (84 percent). However, the cup-shaped N95 with a face mask, cup-shaped N95 with an exhalation valve, PAPR, and cup-shaped N95 with exhalation valve and overlying face mask all had scores significantly lower than the control.

The second set of trials was performed with elastomeric respirators with and without exhalation valves in an audiometric test room with background noise. All six respirators had scores significantly different from the control, and the three respirators with speech augmentation performed better than those without augmentation. The final set of trials was performed in an audiometric test room with background noise with only the listener wearing a PAPR. The PAPR significantly impacted scores (79 percent) compared to the control (90 percent). Intelligibility was higher at 3 feet than at 7 feet, but was not significantly different. Control scores were higher in the audiometric room than in the ICU, possibly due to reverberation and distractions in the ICU area. The authors suggested that respirators should be developed that improve communication among coworkers in noisy medical settings.

Hah and colleagues (2009) investigated loose-fitting PAPRs and N95s for air traffic controllers who would have to work during an influenza pandemic. Although they focused on communications using headsets, some of their observations are applicable to the healthcare environment. The blowers for the three loose-fitting PAPRs that they investigated created noise between 52 dBA and 81 dBA. As expected, the respirator with the highest blower noise had the lowest speech intelligibility scores. Although the authors used a modified rhyme test that was different than the test employed by Radonovich and colleagues (2010), these authors found error rates of 3 to 18 percent with the PAPRs for electronic communications and error rates of 32 to 55 percent with 3 subjects performing face-to-face communications. The quietest PAPR had the lowest error rates. Their N95 tests with two filtering facepiece respirators and one elastomeric respirator had error rates of 0 to 16 percent, though only 2 volunteers were used. The highest errors were with the elastomeric respirator, similar to the Radonovich findings. The elastomeric respirator was rated as obstructing maintenance tasks more than the filtering facepiece respirator.

These three studies showed that background noise, whether it is from a dental drill, ICU room, or PAPR, has a detrimental effect on speech communications. Efforts should be made to decrease ambient noise, select PAPRs with low-noise blowers, or develop and certify PAPRs with lower flow rates that could be used by healthcare personnel. Speech augmentation devices or voice projection units may also improve communications. The Department of Homeland Security has a current Small Business Innovation Research project (Topic Number H-SB09.2-006) (Department of Homeland Security, 2009) that is investigating improved speech intelligibility in noise for first responders. Some of the techniques being developed may be applicable to PAPRs and elastomerics, the respirators that the studies by Radonovich and Hah and colleagues identified as having the greatest decrement on speech recognition. Additionally, the impact of decreased communications on patient care and procedural outcome is unknown.

Current Research Directions

NIOSH recently supported a research effort (Brosseau, 2009) that examined ways to improve fit for half-mask respirators. The effort culminated in a workshop that included presentations on recent research efforts, innovation, design, and impediments to bring new products to market as well as breakout sessions during which participants discussed characteristics of good design, areas where research is needed, wearer characteristics that impact fit, and necessary design changes. Characteristics of good design identified during the breakout session included "low weight, able to fit many facial profiles, does not impair field of vision, uniform pressure on the face, good strap design, can be easily donned multiple times, has a limited number of parts, does not interfere with communication and is portable and easy to store" (Brosseau, 2009, p. 33). Participants identified the following as important research areas: decontaminating respirators, cross-contamination occurrence during repeat donning, efficacy of biocidal coatings, and whether respirator use reduces infection rates in emergency departments. Wearer characteristics that the group identified as contributing to fit were symmetry, chin characteristics, sweat, nose dimension, and head dimension. Participants also identified the need for a user seal check that works and said they would like continuous fit checking rather than a no-fit test. Overarching recommendations for future research were to further investigate the relationship between respirator design and fit; to clarify the impact of facepiece design, facepiece sizes, and aging on the relationship between facial measurements and respirator fit; to determine how user seal check impacts respirator fit; to explore new methods for checking facepiece seals; and to determine the impact of environmental conditions and other protective equipment on respirator fit.

The Department of Veterans Affairs is leading a collaborative effort with the National Personal Protective Technology Laboratory (NPPTL) to develop a respirator specifically designed for healthcare personnel entitled Project Better Respiratory Equipment Using Advanced Technologies for Healthcare Employees (B.R.E.A.T.H.E.) (Department of Veterans Affairs, 2010). The project has been divided into four stages: interagency working group information exchange, prototype development, prototype lab and human subject testing, and commercialization. Nine federal departments and agencies are participating in the working group. The group met in 2008 to discuss issues of safety and effectiveness, impact on occupational activities, comfort and tolerability, and healthcare policies and practices. On December 14, 2009, a notice was placed in the *Federal Register* describing the project and seeking letters of interest from commercial organizations with the ability to design and manufacture a respirator that meets the needs of Project B.R.E.A.T.H.E. (Federal Register, 2009). It is anticipated that the report will be published in 2011.

Summary

Efforts are under way to develop more comfortable and easier to fit respirators that will be more conducive to interactions with patients, colleagues, and family members. Research to date has shown that the low inhalation and exhalation resistance rates of filtering facepiece respirators do not significantly impact respiration. Although hypoventilation occurs with full-facepiece air-purifying respirators, neither the Bansal and colleagues (2009) nor the Roberge and colleagues (2010a,b,c) studies showed any evidence of such a burden with N95 filtering facepiece respirators or elastomeric respirators. Respirators do impact communications. However, the impact of decreased speech intelligibility on task performance is unknown. Loose-fitting PAPRs may make many healthcare tasks more difficult because of their bulkiness, added weight of the blower, flexible visor, and blower noise.

Protective Clothing

Gowns and other forms of protective clothing are designed for healthcare personnel primarily to act as a barrier to prevent the penetration of liquids or solids from coming into contact with the wearer's skin and clothing. As the barrier properties of the protective clothing increase, the breathability of the material generally decreases, which then has the potential to impact comfort and tolerability (i.e., cause an increase in heat levels experienced by the wearer). A recent study has demonstrated that medical personnel who wear chemical protective clothing while performing basic life-saving tasks (e.g., connecting an intravenous [IV] line) experience discomfort and heat stress along with needing more time to perform the task (Rissanen et al., 2008). Using phase-change materials for the construction of protective clothing offers the potential to help reduce heat stress and improve thermal comfort for healthcare personnel.

Phase-change materials provide cooling by absorbing heat when they change from a solid to a liquid state. A surgeon wearing a vest containing phase-change materials reported subjective improvements in thermal comfort over that compared to regular clothing (Reinertsen et al., 2008).

A 2008 review of protective clothing for healthcare personnel highlighted additional issues that are considered in designing protective clothing, including antibacterial finishing treatments, the impact of temperature and relative humidity in the work environment, the use of multiple layers, and changes that can result from laundering or cleaning that might impact the protective effects of the clothing (Laing, 2008). The issue of laundering was further reviewed by Wilson and colleagues (2007), who assessed the limited available literature and found that industrial laundering and home laundering both were effective in decontamination of healthcare clothing, including lab coats.

A large-scale study (Manian and Ponzillo, 2007) examined compliance of gown wear for hospital personnel (n = 1,150) and visitors (n = 392) to general wards and an ICU. Overall compliance by hospital personnel was 76 percent, while visitors complied 65 percent of the time. However, there were differences among healthcare personnel by occupation, with respiratory therapists having the highest compliance rate (96 percent) and physicians having the lowest (67 percent). Female healthcare personnel (79 percent) were more likely than males (66 percent) to wear gowns. Overall compliance was higher in the ICU (83 percent) than in the general wards (71 percent). The study authors did not note whether an individual healthcare professional was included in multiple observations. Additionally, knowing they were being watched may have influenced the decision to wear a gown. The reasons for non-compliance are unknown. However, the study showed that improvement is needed in gown compliance and that educational efforts should focus on male healthcare personnel as well as both healthcare personnel and visitors to general wards.

Gloves

Gloves also serve as barrier protection, although the role of gloves in preventing the transmission of influenza or other respiratory viruses is unknown. For bloodborne pathogens, gloves can prevent transmission through direct contact with non-intact skin. Gloves can provide a barrier between contaminated surfaces and the skin and can serve as a reminder to avoid self-inoculation. However, gloved hands can be a means of self-inoculation if healthcare personnel inadvertently touch their mouth, nose, or eyes with contaminated hands (IOM, 2008). Changing gloves between patients and paying rigorous attention to hand hygiene protocols can reduce contamination between patients or self-inoculation. Glove donning and doffing procedures have been examined to reduce contamination (Jones et al., 2010; Newman et al., 2007).

As with gowns and protective clothing, one active area of research is the use of antiviral coatings or other virus-inhibiting mechanisms. Caillot and Voiglio (2008) examined the tolerance and ease of use of gloves that had a disinfecting agent between the two layers of the glove. They found that tactile feeling, grip quality, and other measures were comparable to double latex gloving. Other areas of study are indicators of perforation in gloves, double gloving, and tolerance of powder or other irritant reducers (e.g., aloe vera) (Fry et al., 2010; Hubner et al., 2010; Korniewicz and El Masri, 2007; Partecke et al., 2009).

Eye Protection and Face Shields

Transmission of influenza through the mucosa of the eyes, nose, and mouth is plausible, but not confirmed (Chan et al., 2010). Case reports of conjunctivitis have been noted with the H7N7 avian influenza virus (Fouchier et al., 2004). Protective eyewear and face shields can reduce self-inoculation and may provide protection against droplet spray. Little is known about how well these devices protect the wearer from direct contact, when this protection is needed regarding transmission from patients to healthcare personnel, and the extent to which extra precautions are needed during aerosol-generating procedures.

Face shields may be a useful form of protection in lieu of face masks for workers exposed to droplet spray, particularly regarding comfort and tolerability issues, reduced breathing resistance, and improved speech communication. Decontamination and reuse may be possible for face shields, but much remains to be learned. It is unknown whether healthcare personnel would find face shields to be an acceptable alternative to masks and whether face shields would provide similar or superior (by protecting the eyes) protection to masks.

The recent literature on eye protection and face shields appears to be limited and focused on blood-splash concerns. A study by Mansour and colleagues (2009) examined eye protection during orthopedic surgery and made comparisons of several types of glasses, loupes, or face shields. Modern prescription glasses offered no benefit over the control condition, with both resulting in contamination rates of 83 percent. These rates were significantly lower for all other eye-protective devices (50 percent for standard surgical telescopic loupes, 30 percent for face-mask and eye-shield combinations, and 3 percent for disposable glasses). Studies have also examined eye protection for blood-splash concerns (Davies et al., 2007; Wines et al., 2008) and found that face masks, eye shields, and glasses worn by surgeons and scrub nurses had high incidence of blood and body-fluid splashes. Similar studies would be useful to evaluate the exposure of healthcare personnel to droplet spray during patient care and to assess which types and combinations of eye protection and face shields provide the greatest protection.

Cross-Cutting Issues: Task Performance and New Materials

Task Performance

The ability of medical staff to perform tasks and medical procedures while wearing PPE is a concern. Several recent studies assessed the impact of various levels of PPE on the ability of healthcare personnel to perform medical tasks. The ability to complete a simulated resuscitation was investigated for paramedics wearing an air-purifying respirator and PAPR (Schumacher et al., 2009) and for paramedics and anesthesia trainees wearing an air-purifying respirator with a binocular or panoramic lens (Brinker et al., 2007; Schumacher et al., 2008). No differences in task completion times were found in any of these three studies. Delays resulting from donning a protective gown were seen in the initiation of chest compressions and cardiopulmonary resuscitation in a study of firefighter defibrillator instructors who were videotaped performing cardiac arrest scenarios (Watson et al., 2008). Rissanen and colleagues (2008) found that completing two medical tasks while wearing chemical, biological, radiological, and nuclear (CBRN) PPE, including an impregnated charcoal suit, overalls, an air-purifying respirator, and cotton and rubber gloves, took longer—19 percent for ventilation and 18 percent for connecting an IV line. Udayasiri and colleagues (2007) assessed the ability of emergency department doctors and nurses to perform trauma resuscitation in level C PPE (air-purifying respirator, hooded suit, and inner and outer gloves) versus gowns and gloves. Although volunteers believed the PPE impaired pulse assessment, IV cannulation, IV-line attachment, mini-jet use, bag and mask ventilation, and communication, only the time to control hemorrhage (38 to 47 sec, $p = 0.02$) was significantly impacted. Castle and colleagues (2009) assessed the ability of 64 clinicians to perform intubation, laryngeal mask airway placement, and insertion of an IV cannula and intraosseous needle twice while in CBRN PPE and once unsuited. Eight percent of intubation and 12 percent of IV cannulation attempts were unsuccessful in CBRN PPE.

Donning of PPE has also been noted to delay the onset of patient care. Watson and colleagues (2009) conducted a simulation of a patient on a pediatric ward who developed respiratory failure. Donning of full PPE delayed the first response to the simulated "code" situation by 2 minutes, and other care measures were also delayed.

These results show that many medical tasks can be performed in various levels of PPE, but that the tasks may take longer. No studies were performed that assessed the impact of filtering facepiece respirators, elastomeric respirators, or loose-fitting PAPRs on task performance. However, a filtering facepiece respirator or elastomeric respirator is unlikely to have a greater impact on task performance than a full-facepiece air-purifying respirator. The bulkiness and visor of a loose-fitting PAPR may have a different impact on performance than the more close-fitting air-purifying respirator and PAPR used in these studies. Castle and colleagues (2009) report that the reason some tasks could not be completed may be because clinicians were wearing full chemical, biological suits. The individual impact of respirators, suits, and rubber gloves cannot be separated. Additional studies that assess the impact on task performance of PPE likely to be worn during an influenza pandemic or outbreak of other viral respiratory diseases are warranted.

Using Multiple Types of PPE: Integration and Use Issues

Because healthcare personnel frequently need to use several PPE items for protection against bloodborne or other infectious agents, including a respirator, gloves, a gown, eye or face protection, and in some cases head and shoe coverings, issues arise about the integration and interface of these items and how best to don and doff the PPE to ensure that maximum protection is provided and contamination is avoided. Workers in fields such as law enforcement, firefighting, and health care have critical needs to be able to perform specific tasks while wearing multiple types and models of PPE. The impact of PPE on occupation-specific tasks and the equipment used to perform those tasks should be considered in designing and selecting PPE.

Studies on the impact of PPE on medical tasks have focused on chemical and biological protective equipment (Brinker et al., 2007; Castle et al., 2009; Rissanen et al., 2008; Schumacher et al., 2008, 2009; Udayasiri et al., 2007). These studies did not address healthcare-specific PPE used to protect against influenza transmission. The impact of individual PPE items was not assessed, so it is not known whether the respirator, gloves, or suits or a combination of equipment caused the interference. Additionally, face shields were not used in these studies. Integration of common healthcare PPE with medical equipment should be assessed and their impact on task performance determined.

SUMMARY OF PROGRESS

Personal protective equipment is a critical component in the hierarchy of controls used to protect healthcare personnel from influenza and other viral respiratory diseases. Understanding the functional issues related to the design of PPE as well as the factors that impact use are critical to ensuring that healthcare personnel are adequately protected, comfortable, and able to perform their jobs. Important advances have been made in some areas since the 2008 IOM report, but other areas, particularly regarding improvements in gowns, gloves, face masks, and face shields, need to be more fully addressed. Much research has been done regarding filtration of respirator media, but ways to improve fit, including new technologies specifically for filtering facepiece respirators, need more research because face seal leakage greatly exceeds filter penetration in the overall TIL of respirators. The physiological impact of respirators has been studied in-depth, but research in this area is lacking for other types of PPE. Integration issues concerning PPE and medical equipment and the impact on operational performance have not been adequately studied. Effective decontamination methods that do not impact the physical characteristics of respirators have been studied for some types of respirators, but with inconclusive results. Finally, the characteristics of a respirator that would specifically address the needs of healthcare personnel (e.g., patient–provider interaction, comfort, reduced physiological burden) have been identified. Addressing these issues is important for developing PPE for healthcare personnel that is safe, effective, and comfortable.

FINDINGS AND RESEARCH NEEDS

This chapter provides an overview of the range of ongoing work on designing and engineering effective PPE to prevent transmission of influenza and other viral respiratory diseases. At its June 2010 workshop and through its literature review, the committee realized that many research efforts have been completed recently and that ongoing research efforts in this area continue. The challenge will be to sustain these efforts and to broaden them into areas that will result in wearable and effective PPE for healthcare personnel. Box 3-1 highlights the committee's findings in this area.

- **Wearability:**

  - *Respirators:* Continue examining the features of N95s, PAPRs, and elastomeric respirators that impact comfort and tolerability among healthcare personnel. Identify alterations in respirator design and construction that show promise in improving problem features that adversely impact comfort and tolerability.
  - *Other PPE:* Initiate research to identify factors affecting the comfort and tolerability of protective eyewear and clothing, and identify changes having the potential to positively influence comfort and tolerability. Evaluate differences between short- and long-term use of PPE as it affects comfort and tolerability. Develop and field test new designs and features for PPE for healthcare personnel that offer potential for improving comfort and tolerability.

- **Decontamination and Feasibility of Reuse:**

  - *Decontamination methods:* Continue to assess promising decontamination methods for all types of PPE, including research on the impact of decontamination methods on respirator protection and on the physical characteristics of

---

BOX 3-1
Findings

- Respirators are designed to provide respiratory protection, and respirators certified by the National Institute for Occupational Safety and Health are tested to provide effective filtration. Issues remain regarding respirator fit, which currently depends on fit testing and user seal checks. Efforts focused on addressing total inward leakage may resolve some of these issues, and research on respirators that do not require fit testing is needed.
- Face masks and face shields do not provide a tight seal to the wearer's face. Laboratory research to date on the performance of face masks has focused on inhalable particulates, and there has been little or no research as to the performance of these devices on droplet spray.
- There is a lack of knowledge as to the performance of eye protection, face shields, gloves and gowns, and other PPE in protecting the wearer from influenza and other respiratory viruses.

---

the respirator (inner, middle, and outer layers). Assess decontamination effectiveness using either influenza virus or a suitable surrogate.

o *Feasibility of reuse:* Develop a protocol for donning and doffing PPE to minimize self-inoculation.

- **TIL and Protection:**

  o *TIL:* Finish development of the TIL certification requirements for half-mask air-purifying respirators. Assess TIL of very small particles (< 100 nm) with respirators.

  o *Face masks and face shields:* Assess the TIL of face masks against droplet spray. Conduct research using manned and unmanned tests to determine if face shields can offer suitable alternative protection to goggles and/or face masks to protect healthcare personnel against droplet spray.

  o *Fit:* Evaluate the impact of facepiece materials and design on improving the fit of filtering facepiece respirators. Develop improved and simpler fit testing methods. Examine the effectiveness of performing a user seal check for an N95 respirator each time it is donned.

  o *Workplace protection studies:* Conduct workplace protection studies to assess protection during typical tasks and time changes in protection. Determine how using typical instruments impacts protection, and identify integration issues.

- **Equipment and Technologies:**

  o *Integration:* Conduct human factors (field of view, visual acuity, communication) and operational performance studies to assess the ability of healthcare personnel to perform medical procedures in typical healthcare-specific PPE ensembles.
  o *New technologies:* Continue development of an air-purifying respirator that specifically addresses the needs of healthcare personnel. New materials and technologies should be developed specifically for filtering facepiece respirators to improve fit, comfort, and tolerability. A new low-noise, lightweight, PAPR and a face shield that is reusable and easy to clean should be designed and developed. The efficacy and effectiveness of antiviral-coated PPE and impacts on maintenance and reuse of PPE should be assessed.

RECOMMENDATIONS

Recommendation: <u>Continue and Expand Research on PPE for Healthcare Personnel</u>
NPPTL and other agencies, private-sector companies, and other organizations should continue to advance research in designing and evaluating the effectiveness of respirator protection for healthcare personnel and expand its research efforts to improve and evaluate the effectiveness of gloves, gowns, eye protection, face shields, and face masks in preventing the transmission of influenza or other viral respiratory diseases. Areas of focused research needs include

- **effectiveness in preventing fomite, droplet spray, or aerosol transmission;**
- **decontamination and feasibility of reuse;**
- **comfort, fit, and usability;**
- **impact on task performance; and**
- **development of technologies specifically for healthcare personnel.**

Recommendation: <u>Improve Fit Test Methods and Evaluate</u> <u>User Seal Checks</u>
NPPTL should develop novel, simpler fit test methods and evaluate the effectiveness of performing user seal checks on N95 respirators.

Recommendation: <u>Develop and Certify PAPRs for Health-</u> <u>care Personnel</u>
NPPTL should develop certification requirements for a low-noise, loose-fitting PAPR for healthcare personnel.

Recommendation: <u>Examine the Effectiveness of Face Masks</u> <u>and Face Shields as PPE</u>
NPPTL should investigate the effectiveness of face masks and face shields in preventing transmission of viral respiratory diseases.

REFERENCES

Au, S. S., C. D. Gomersall, P. Leung, and P. T. Li. 2010. A randomised controlled pilot study to compare filtration factor of a novel non-fit-tested high-efficiency particulate air (HEPA) filtering facemask with a fit-tested N95 mask. *Journal of Hospital Infection* 76(1):23-25.

Baig, A. S., C. Knapp, A. E. Eagan, and L. J. Radonovich, Jr. 2010. Health care workers' views about respirator use and features that should be included in the next generation of respirators. *American Journal of Infection Control* 38(1):18-25.

Bansal, S., P. Harber, D. Yun, D. Liu, Y. Liu, S. Wu, D. Ng, and S. Santiago. 2009. Respirator physiological effects under simulated work conditions. *Journal of Occupational and Environmental Hygiene* 6(4):221-227.

Borkow, G., S. S. Zhou, T. Page, and J. Gabbay. 2010. A novel anti-influenza copper oxide containing respiratory face mask. *PLoS ONE* 5(6):e11295.

Brinker, A., S. A. Gray, and J. Schumacher. 2007. Influence of air-purifying respirators on the simulated first response emergency treatment of CBRN victims. *Resuscitation* 74(2):310-316.

Brosseau, L. M. 2009. *Toward better fitting respirators: No fit test respirator workshop and research roadmap, RFQ 2008-Q-10205.* http://www.sph. umn.edu/ce/presentations/docs/Final_NoFitRespiratorReport_July28_2009. pdf (accessed November 30, 2010).

Brosseau, L. M., and K. Harriman. 2007. Commentary on "in vivo protective performance of N95 respirator and surgical facemask." *American Journal of Industrial Medicine* 50(12):1025-1026; author reply 1027-1029.

Caillot, J. L., and E. J. Voiglio. 2008. First clinical study of a new virus-inhibiting surgical glove. *Swiss Medical Weekly* 138(1-2):18-22.

Casanova, L., W. A. Rutala, D. J. Weber, and M. D. Sobsey. 2009. Methods for the recovery of a model virus from healthcare personal protective equipment. *Journal of Applied Microbiology* 106(4):1244-1251.

Castle, N., R. Owen, M. Hann, S. Clark, D. Reeves, and I. Gurney. 2009. Impact of chemical, biological, radiation, and nuclear personal protective equipment on the performance of low- and high-dexterity airway and vascular access skills. *Resuscitation* 80(11):1290-1295.

Chan, M. C., R. W. Chan, W. C. Yu, C. C. Ho, K. M. Yuen, J. H. Fong, L. L. Tang, W. W. Lai, A. C. Lo, W. H. Chui, A. D. Sihoe, D. L. Kwong, D. S. Wong, G. S. Tsao, L. L. Poon, Y. Guan, J. M. Nicholls, and J. S. Peiris. 2010. Tropism and innate host responses of the 2009 pandemic H1N1 influenza virus in ex vivo and in vitro cultures of human conjunctiva and respiratory tract. *American Journal of Pathology* 176(4):1828-1840.

Cho, K. J., T. Reponen, R. McKay, R. Shukla, H. Haruta, P. Sekar, and S. A. Grinshpun. 2010. Large particle penetration through N95 respirator filters and facepiece leaks with cyclic flow. *Annals of Occupational Hygiene* 54(1):68-77.

Coffey, C. C., R. B. Lawrence, D. L. Campbell, Z. Zhuang, C. A. Calvert, and P. A. Jensen. 2004. Fitting characteristics of eighteen N95 filtering-facepiece respirators. *Journal of Occupational and Environmental Hygiene* 1(4):262-271.

Davies, C. G., M. N. Khan, A. S. Ghauri, and C. J. Ranaboldo. 2007. Blood and body fluid splashes during surgery—the need for eye protection and masks. *Annals of the Royal College of Surgeons of England* 89(8):770-772.

Department of Homeland Security. 2009. *Noise cancellation for voice operated switch (VOX) communications: Small Business Innovation Research project topic number H-SB09.2-006.* https://www.sbir.dhs.gov/reference/DHS_SBIR-2009.2_Full_Solicitation.doc (accessed November 4, 2010).

Department of Veterans Affairs. 2010. *National Center for Occupational Health and Infection Control: Key projects.* http://www.publichealth.va.gov/employeehealth/epidemiccontrol/projects.asp#breathe (accessed November 4, 2010).

Diaz, K. T., and G. C. Smaldone. 2010. Quantifying exposure risk: Surgical masks and respirators. *American Journal of Infection Control* 38(7):501-508.

Duling, M. G., R. B. Lawrence, J. E. Slaven, and C. C. Coffey. 2007. Simulated workplace protection factors for half-facepiece respiratory protective devices. *Journal of Occupational and Environmental Hygiene* 4(6):420-431.

Eninger, R. M., T. Honda, A. Adhikari, H. Heinonen-Tanski, T. Reponen, and S. A. Grinshpun. 2008a. Filter performance of N99 and N95 facepiece respirators against viruses and ultrafine particles. *Annals of Occupational Hygiene* 52(5):385-396.

Eninger, R. M., T. Honda, T. Reponen, R. McKay, and S. A. Grinshpun. 2008b. What does respirator certification tell us about filtration of ultrafine particles? *Journal of Occupational and Environmental Hygiene* 5(5):286-295.

Eshbaugh, J. P., P. D. Gardner, A. W. Richardson, and K. C. Hofacre. 2009. N95 and P100 respirator filter efficiency under high constant and cyclic flow. *Journal of Occupational and Environmental Hygiene* 6(1):52-61.

Federal Register. 2009. *Notice: Department of Veterans Affairs: Project Better Respiratory Equipment Using Advanced Technologies for Healthcare Employees (B.R.E.A.T.H.E.).* http://frwebgate3.access.gpo.gov/cgi-bin/PDF gate.cgi?WAISdocID=ceFTAw/1/2/0&WAISaction=retrieve (accessed November 4, 2010).

Fisher, E., and R. Shaffer. 2010. Survival of bacteriophage MS2 on filtering facepiece respirator coupons. *Applied Biosafety* 15(2):71-76.

Fisher, E., S. Rengasamy, D. Viscusi, E. Vo, and R. Shaffer. 2009. Development of a test system to apply virus-containing particles to filtering facepiece respirators for the evaluation of decontamination procedures. *Applied and Environmental Microbiology* 75(6):1500-1507.

Fouchier, R. A. M., P. M. Schneeberger, F. W. Rozendaal, J. M. Broekman, S. A. G. Kemink, V. Munster, T. Kuiken, G. F. Rimmelzwaan, M. Schutten, G. J. J. van Doornum, G. Koch, A. Bosman, M. Koopmans, and A. D. M. E. Osterhaus. 2004. Avian influenza A virus (H7N7) associated with human conjunctivitis and a fatal case of acute respiratory distress syndrome. *Proceedings of the National Academy of Sciences (U.S.A.)* 101(5):1356-1361.

Fry, D. E., W. E. Harris, E. N. Kohnke, and C. L. Twomey. 2010. Influence of double-gloving on manual dexterity and tactile sensation of surgeons. *Journal of the American College of Surgeons* 210(3):325-330.

Grinshpun, S. A., H. Haruta, R. M. Eninger, T. Reponen, R. T. McKay, and S. A. Lee. 2009. Performance of an N95 filtering facepiece particulate respirator and a surgical mask during human breathing: Two pathways for particle penetration. *Journal of Occupational and Environmental Hygiene* 6(10):593-603.

Hah, S., T. Yuditsky, K. A. Schulz, H. Dorsey, A. R. Deshmukh, and J. Sharra. 2009. *Evaluation of human performance while wearing respirators.* http://hf.tc.faa.gov/technotes/dot-faa-tc-09-10.pdf (accessed November 3, 2010).

Harber, P., S. Bansal, S. Santiago, D. Liu, D. Yun, D. Ng, Y. Liu, and S. Wu. 2009. Multidomain subjective response to respirator use during simulated work. *Journal of Occupational and Environmental Medicine* 51(1):38-45.

Heimbuch, B. K., K. Kinney, B. Nichols, and J. D. Wander. 2009. The dry aerosol deposition device (DADD): An instrument for depositing microbial aerosols onto surfaces. *Journal of Microbiological Methods* 78(3):255-259.

Huang, J. T., and V. I. Huang. 2007. Evaluation of the efficiency of medical masks and the creation of new medical masks. *Journal of International Medical Research* 35(2):213-223.

Hubner, N. O., A. M. Goerdt, N. Stanislawski, O. Assadian, C. D. Heidecke, A. Kramer, and L. I. Partecke. 2010. Bacterial migration through punctured surgical gloves under real surgical conditions. *BMC Infectious Diseases* 10:192.

IOM (Institute of Medicine). 2008. *Preparing for an influenza pandemic: Personal protective equipment for healthcare workers.* Washington, DC: The National Academies Press.

Janssen, L. L., T. J. Nelson, and K. T. Cuta. 2007. Workplace protection factors for an N95 filtering facepiece respirator. *Journal of Occupational and Environmental Hygiene* 4(9):698-707.

Johnson, A. T., F. C. Koh, S. Jamshidi, and T. E. Rehak. 2008. Human subject testing of leakage in a loose-fitting papr. *Journal of Occupational and Environmental Hygiene* 5(5):325-329.

Johnson, D. F., J. D. Druce, C. Birch, and M. L. Grayson. 2009. A quantitative assessment of the efficacy of surgical and N95 masks to filter influenza virus in patients with acute influenza infection. *Clinical Infectious Diseases* 49(2):275-277.

Jones, C., B. Brooker, and M. Genon. 2010. Comparison of open and closed staff-assisted glove donning on the nature of surgical glove cuff contamination. *Australian and New Zealand Journal of Surgery* 80(3):174-177.

Korniewicz, D. M., and M. El Masri. 2007. Effect of aloe-vera impregnated gloves on hand hygiene attitudes of health care workers. *MEDSURG Nursing* 16(4):247-252.

Laing, R. M. 2008. Protection provided by clothing and textiles against potential hazards in the operating theatre. *International Journal of Occupational and Safety Ergonomics* 14(1):107-115.

Lee, J. H., C. Y. Wu, K. M. Wysocki, S. Farrah, and J. Wander. 2008a. Efficacy of iodine-treated biocidal filter media against bacterial spore aerosols. *Journal of Applied Microbiology* 105(5):1318-1326.

Lee, J. H., C. Y. Wu, C. N. Lee, D. Anwar, K. M. Wysocki, D. A. Lundgren, S. Farrah, J. Wander, and B. K. Heimbuch. 2009. Assessment of iodine-treated filter media for removal and inactivation of MS2 bacteriophage aerosols. *Journal of Applied Microbiology* 107(6):1912-1923.

Lee, M. C., S. Takaya, R. Long, and A. M. Joffe. 2008b. Respirator-fit testing: Does it ensure the protection of healthcare workers against respirable particles carrying pathogens? *Infection Control and Hospital Epidemiology* 29(12):1149-1156.

Lee, S. A., S. A. Grinshpun, and T. Reponen. 2008c. Respiratory performance offered by N95 respirators and surgical masks: Human subject evaluation with NaCl aerosol representing bacterial and viral particle size range. *Annals of Occupational Hygiene* 52(3):177-185.

Li, Y., T. Wong, J. Chung, Y. P. Guo, J. Y. Hu, Y. T. Guan, L. Yao, Q. W. Song, and E. Newton. 2006. In vivo protective performance of N95 respirator and surgical facemask. *American Journal of Industrial Medicine* 49(12):1056-1065.

Manian, F. A., and J. J. Ponzillo. 2007. Compliance with routine use of gowns by healthcare workers (HCWs) and non-HCW visitors on entry into the rooms of patients under contact precautions. *Infection Control and Hospital Epidemiology* 28(3):337-340.

Mansour, A. A., 3rd, J. L. Even, S. Phillips, and J. L. Halpern. 2009. Eye protection in orthopaedic surgery. An in vitro study of various forms of eye protection and their effectiveness. *Journal of Bone and Joint Surgery* 91(5):1050-1054.

McMahon, E., K. Wada, and A. Dufresne. 2008. Implementing fit testing for N95 filtering facepiece respirators: Practical information from a large cohort of hospital workers. *American Journal of Infection Control* 36(4):298-300.

Mendel, L. L., J. A. Gardino, and S. R. Atcherson. 2008. Speech understanding using surgical masks: A problem in health care? *Journal of the American Academy of Audiology* 19(9):686-695.

Monaghan, W. D., M. R. Roberge, M. Rengasamy, and R. J. Roberge. 2009. Thermal imaging comparison of maximum surface temperatures achieved on N95 filtering facepiece respirators with and without exhalation valves at sedentary breathing volumes. *Journal of the International Society for Respiratory Protection* 26:12-19.

Newman, J. B., M. Bullock, and R. Goyal. 2007. Comparison of glove donning techniques for the likelihood of gown contamination. An infection control study. *Acta Orthopaedica Belgica* 73(6):765-771.

Oberg, T., and L. M. Brosseau. 2008. Surgical mask filter and fit performance. *American Journal of Infection Control* 36(4):276-282.

Oestenstad, R. K., and A. A. Bartolucci. 2010. Factors affecting the location and shape of face seal leak sites on half-mask respirators. *Journal of Occupational and Environmental Hygiene* 7(6):332-341.

Oestenstad, R. K., L. J. Elliott, and T. M. Beasley. 2007. The effect of gender and respirator brand on the association of respirator fit with facial dimensions. *Journal of Occupational and Environmental Hygiene* 4(12):923-930.

Oxford, J. S., R. Lambkin, M. Guralnik, R. A. Rosenbloom, M. P. Petteruti, K. Digian, and C. Lefante. 2007. Preclinical in vitro activity of QR-435 against influenza A virus as a virucide and in paper masks for prevention of viral transmission. *American Journal of Therapeutics* 14(5):455-461.

Partecke, L. I., A. M. Goerdt, I. Langner, B. Jaeger, O. Assadian, C. D. Heidecke, A. Kramer, and N. O. Huebner. 2009. Incidence of microperforation for surgical gloves depends on duration of wear. *Infection Control and Hospital Epidemiology* 30(5):409-414.

Radonovich, L. J., Jr., J. Cheng, B. V. Shenal, M. Hodgson, and B. S. Bender. 2009. Respirator tolerance in health care workers. *Journal of the American Medical Association* 301(1):36-38.

Radonovich, L. J., Jr., R. Yanke, J. Cheng, and B. Bender. 2010. Diminished speech intelligibility associated with certain types of respirators worn by healthcare workers. *Journal of Occupational and Environmental Hygiene* 7(1):63-70.

Reinertsen, R. E., H. Faerevik, K. Holbo, R. Nesbakken, J. Reitan, A. Royset, and M. Suong Le Thi. 2008. Optimizing the performance of phase-change materials in personal protective clothing systems. *International Journal of Occupational Safety and Ergonomics* 14(1):43-53.

Rengasamy, S., W. P. King, B. C. Eimer, and R. E. Shaffer. 2008. Filtration performance of NIOSH-approved N95 and P100 filtering facepiece respirators against 4 to 30 nanometer-size nanoparticles. *Journal of Occupational and Environmental Hygiene* 5(9):556-564.

Rengasamy, S., B. C. Eimer, and R. E. Shaffer. 2009. Comparison of nanoparticle filtration performance of NIOSH-approved and CE-marked particulate filtering facepiece respirators. *Annals of Occupational Hygiene* 53(2):117-128.

Rengasamy, S., B. Eimer, and R. E. Shaffer. 2010a. Simple respiratory protection—evaluation of the filtration performance of cloth masks and common fabric materials against 20-1000 nm size particles. *Annals of Occupational Hygiene* 54(7):789-798.

Rengasamy, S., E. Fisher, and R. E. Shaffer. 2010b. Evaluation of the survivability of MS2 viral aerosols deposited on filtering face piece respirator samples incorporating antimicrobial technologies. *American Journal of Infection Control* 38(1):9-17.

Rissanen, S., I. Jousela, J. R. Jeong, and H. Rintamaki. 2008. Heat stress and bulkiness of chemical protective clothing impair performance of medical personnel in basic lifesaving tasks. *Ergonomics* 51(7):1011-1022.

Roberge, M. R., M. R. Vojtko, R. J. Roberge, R. J. Vojtko, and D. P. Landsittel. 2008. Wearing an N95 respirator concurrently with a powered air-purifying respirator: Effect on protection factor. *Respiratory Care* 53(12):1685-1690.

Roberge, R. J. 2008. Evaluation of the rationale for concurrent use of N95 filtering facepiece respirators with loose-fitting powered air-purifying respirators during aerosol-generating medical procedures. *American Journal of Infection Control* 36(2):135-141.

———. 2009. Physiological burden associated with the use of filtering facepiece respirators (N95 masks) during pregnancy. *Journal of Women's Health* 18(6):819-826.

Roberge, R. J., A. Coca, W. J. Williams, A. J. Palmiero, and J. B. Powell. 2010a. Surgical mask placement over N95 filtering facepiece respirators: Physiological effects on healthcare workers. *Respirology* 15(3):516-521.

Roberge, R. J., A. Coca, W. J. Williams, J. B. Powell, and A. J. Palmiero. 2010b. Physiological impact of the N95 filtering facepiece respirator on healthcare workers. *Respiratory Care* 55(5):569-577.

———. 2010c. Reusable elastomeric air-purifying respirators: Physiologic impact on health care workers. *American Journal of Infection Control* 38(5):381-386.

Salter, W. B., K. Kinney, W. H. Wallace, A. E. Lumley, B. K. Heimbuch, and J. D. Wander. 2010. Analysis of residual chemicals on filtering facepiece respirators after decontamination. *Journal of Occupational and Environmental Hygiene* 7(8):437-445.

Schumacher, J., J. Runte, A. Brinker, K. Prior, M. Heringlake, and W. Eichler. 2008. Respiratory protection during high-fidelity simulated resuscitation of casualties contaminated with chemical warfare agents. *Anaesthesia* 63(6):593-598.

Schumacher, J., S. A. Gray, L. Weidelt, A. Brinker, K. Prior, and W. M. Stratling. 2009. Comparison of powered and conventional air-purifying respirators during simulated resuscitation of casualties contaminated with hazardous substances. *Emergency Medicine Journal* 26(7):501-505.

Shaffer, R., and S. Rengasamy. 2009. Respiratory protection against airborne nanoparticles: A review. *Journal of Nanoparticle Research* 11(7):1661-1672.

Tang, J. W., T. J. Liebner, B. A. Craven, and G. S. Settles. 2009. A schlieren optical study of the human cough with and without wearing masks for aerosol infection control. *Journal of the Royal Society Interface* 6(Suppl. 6):S727-S736.

Udayasiri, R., J. Knott, D. T. D. Mc, J. Papson, F. Leow, and F. A. Hassan. 2007. Emergency department staff can effectively resuscitate in level C personal protective equipment. *Emergency Medicine in Australasia* 19(2):113-121.

Viscusi, D., W. King, and R. Shaffer. 2007. Effect of decontamination on the filtration efficiency of two FFR models. *Journal of the International Society for Respiratory Protection* 24:93-107.

Viscusi, D. J., M. Bergman, E. Sinkule, and R. E. Shaffer. 2009a. Evaluation of the filtration performance of 21 N95 filtering face piece respirators after prolonged storage. *American Journal of Infection Control* 37(5):381-386.

Viscusi, D. J., M. S. Bergman, B. C. Eimer, and R. E. Shaffer. 2009b. Evaluation of five decontamination methods for filtering facepiece respirators. *Annals of Occupational Hygiene* 53(8):815-827.

Vo, E., S. Rengasamy, and R. Shaffer. 2009. Development of a test system to evaluate procedures for decontamination of respirators containing viral droplets. *Applied and Environmental Microbiology* 75(23):7303-7309.

Vojtko, M. R., M. R. Roberge, R. J. Vojtko, R. J. Roberge, and D. P. Landsittel. 2008. Effect on breathing resistance of a surgical mask worn over a N95 filtering facepiece respirator. *Journal of the International Society for Respiratory Protection* 25:1-8.

Wander, J., and B. Heimbuch. 2009. *Challenge of N95 and P100 filtering facepiece respirators with particle containing viable H1N1.* Pittsburgh, PA: National Institute for Occupational Safety and Health.

Watson, C. M., M. C. McCrory, J. M. Duval-Arnould, and E. A. Hunt. 2009. Abstract P212: Simulated pediatric resuscitation during novel H1N1 influenza outbreak. *Circulation* 120:S1487-S1488.

Watson, L., W. Sault, R. Gwyn, and P. R. Verbeek. 2008. The "delay effect" of donning a gown during cardiopulmonary resuscitation in a simulation model. *Canadian Journal of Emergency Medical Care* 10(4):333-338.

Wilkinson, I. J., D. Pisaniello, J. Ahmad, and S. Edwards. 2010. Evaluation of a large-scale quantitative respirator-fit testing program for healthcare workers: Survey results. *Infection Control and Hospital Epidemiology* 31(9):918-925.

Wilson, J. A., H. P. Loveday, P. N. Hoffman, and R. J. Pratt. 2007. Uniform: An evidence review of the microbiological significance of uniforms and uniform policy in the prevention and control of healthcare-associated infections. Report to the Department of Health (England). *Journal of Hospital Infection* 66(4):301-307.

Wines, M. P., A. Lamb, A. N. Argyropoulos, A. Caviezel, C. Ganncliffe, and D. Tolley. 2008. Blood splash injury: An underestimated risk in endourology. *Journal of Endourology* 22(6):1183-1187.

Winter, S., J. H. Thomas, D. P. Stephens, and J. S. Davis. 2010. Particulate face masks for protection against airborne pathogens—one size does not fit all: An observational study. *Critical Care and Resuscitation* 12(1):24-27.

Zhuang, Z., B. Bradtmiller, and R. E. Shaffer. 2007. New respirator fit test panels representing the current U.S. civilian work force. *Journal of Occupational and Environmental Hygiene* 4(9):647-659.

Zhuang, Z., D. Groce, H. W. Ahlers, W. Iskander, D. Landsittel, S. Guffey, S. Benson, D. Viscusi, and R. E. Shaffer. 2008. Correlation between respirator fit and respirator fit test panel cells by respirator size. *Journal of Occupational and Environmental Hygiene* 5(10):617-628.

4

Using PPE:
Individual and Organizational Issues

Workers in a wide range of industries are required to wear personal protective equipment (PPE) to reduce or prevent exposures to hazardous chemicals, fire, particulates, or other health risks. As noted in Chapter 3, researchers, designers, and manufacturers continue to look for improvements to the equipment that can reduce the physiological burdens, improve communication, and be more comfortable and less of an encumbrance to wear. For healthcare personnel, the trade-offs of hazardous exposures with the challenges of donning, wearing, and doffing PPE often end up with healthcare personnel not fully adhering to PPE and infection control protocols. This chapter focuses on what has been learned about use of PPE by healthcare personnel and efforts to improve the safety culture in healthcare facilities. The chapter concludes with recommendations for future research.

BACKGROUND AND CONTEXT FROM THE 2008 REPORT

Although healthcare personnel often face hazardous working conditions with potential exposures to a variety of toxic and infectious agents, adherence to PPE protocols is often quite low. Observational studies and survey questionnaires of individual workers have looked at the reasons for the noncompliance and barriers to use, which often include the host of comfort and workability issues discussed in Chapter 3. Few studies have tested interventions to improve adherence rates.

The range of factors that impact PPE-related behaviors and compliance were organized in the 2008 Institute of Medicine (IOM) report and in other studies into three categories:

1. individual factors, such as knowledge, beliefs, attitudes, perception of risk, history, and sociodemographics;
2. environmental factors, including availability of equipment and negative-pressure rooms; and
3. organizational factors, such as management's expectations and performance feedback, workplace policies, and training and education programs.

Discussion in the 2008 report focused on the concerted efforts needed by individual healthcare personnel, managers, and institutions to improve the safety culture in healthcare facilities. This culture requires "an organization-wide dedication to the creation, implementation, evaluation, and maintenance of effective and current safety practices" (IOM, 2008, p. 8). Although organizational and cultural factors in the context of patient safety have received a great deal of attention in recent years, less attention has been focused on healthcare worker safety. In industrial settings, such as chemical and power plants, a focus on achieving high safety performance has been found to result from a sustained emphasis on safety factors at all levels of the organization: the individual level (e.g., attitudes, training), microorganizational level (e.g., management support, safety representatives, accountability), and macroorganizational level (e.g., communication, organization of technology, work processes) (Hofmann et al., 1995). Much can be learned from "high-reliability organizations" (e.g., nuclear power industry; certain military operations, including aircraft carriers; commercial aviation), which are given that term because of their highly complex and hazardous missions and few safety-related failures. Characteristics of these organizations include commitment to safety articulated from the highest level of the organization; resources, incentives, and rewards to carry out the commitment; continuous emphasis on safety; safety as the priority even at the expense of production or efficiency; communication across all levels that is frequent and candid; openness about errors and issues as well as regular reporting; and valuing organizational learning and improvements (Gaba et al., 2003; Roberts, 1990; Rochlin, 1999; Singer et al., 2003; Weick et al., 1999). In many industrial work situations PPE use is considered a mandatory practice with a specific type of PPE or PPE ensemble required whenever a certain job or task is performed. In health care, PPE use is often indicated for certain tasks, but often only under certain conditions.

Implementing a culture of safety can require changes in the organization's policies, procedures, managerial actions and priorities, and resources dedicated to safety with access to effective safety equipment. Furthermore, the commitment to, and support of, safety is conveyed to workers at all levels through active and sincere engagement by those in leadership positions who model, encourage, and enforce appropriate PPE use and safety. Finally, and importantly, individual accountability is key to improving and sustaining PPE use.

The 2008 report identified four key factors in promoting a culture of safety within healthcare facilities; factors where research is still needed to improve PPE adherence are as follows:

1. **Provide leadership, commitment, and role modeling for worker safety:** Employees who perceive a strong organization-wide commitment to safety have been found to be more than 2.5 times more likely to adhere to safety protocols than those who lack such perceptions (Gershon et al., 1995).
2. **Emphasize healthcare worker education and training:** The presence of safety education within a hospital or other healthcare facility demonstrates the organization's commitment to safety and increases individual knowledge of safety practices.
3. **Improve feedback and enforcement of PPE policies and use:** The purpose of developing a positive and strong culture of safety in the workplace is to promote habitual safety practice. As noted in the IOM report,

> Employees should feel *uncomfortable* when *not* wearing PPE during appropriate situations, and supervisors should reinforce the importance of PPE and enforce policies so that noncompliance is the rare exception and not the rule. . . . Each healthcare employer should assume responsibility for taking an active role in facilitating, promoting, and requiring safety actions. Healthcare facilities need to foster and promote a strong culture of safety that includes a commitment to worker safety, adequate access to safety equipment, and extensive training efforts that utilize protocols requiring specific safety actions and detailing consequences for noncompliance. (IOM, 2008, p. 8)

4. **Clarify worksite practices and policies:** Much remains to be learned about specific issues related to wearing PPE in the healthcare setting, particularly during an influenza pandemic. A concerted effort to identify best practices in infection control and to disseminate this information to other healthcare facilities could increase worker and patient safety and have positive ramifications well beyond preparedness for an influenza pandemic.

As noted throughout the prior report, the use of PPE is only one component of promoting a strong safety culture in healthcare settings. In addition to PPE, the continuum of infection prevention and safety controls includes environmental and engineering controls (e.g., number of air exchanges, availability of isolation rooms with negative-pressure ventilation) and administrative or work practice controls (e.g., protocols to ensure early disease recognition, vaccination policies, infection control guidelines for patients and visitors).

UPDATE ON RECENT RESEARCH

Organizational Factors Influencing Use of PPE

In healthcare organizations much of the emphasis on safety in the past decade has focused on patient safety (IOM, 2000). The relationship between patient safety and worker safety is beginning to be further explored, and research continues into delineating the role of a number of factors in creating and sustaining a culture of safety in the healthcare workplace (Lowe, 2008; Singer et al., 2009; Tucker et al., 2008). High-hazard industries, such as commercial aviation and nuclear power, are a major source for research on safety culture and provide useful information to mitigate hazard risk. For example, Lombardi and colleagues (2009) conducted a series of focus group discussions with 51 personnel—primarily from manufacturing, construction, and retail industries as well as a few in health care—on the use of protective eyewear. The authors reported that risk perception, barriers to use of PPE, and enforcement and reinforcement are important safety culture concepts. Investigators further indicated that safety culture emerged as an important theme in encouraging PPE use, which included proper training, personal responsibility, peer pressure to use PPE, and appropriate and comfortable equipment. Supervisor and peer use of PPE was deemed important. As noted by

Lombardi and colleagues, "If the supervisor doesn't have [protective eyewear] on, no one else is going to wear them" (2009, p. 758). Positive reinforcement was seen as encouraging; however, personnel often reported negative reinforcement by supervisors, such as being written up or threatened with job loss. Without enforcement, personnel questioned management's sincerity about safety.

A recent experimental study of social modeling of PPE use found a moderate positive correlation in the number of participants wearing PPE (hearing protection in this study) and the number of safety model peers who wore the hearing protection (Olson et al., 2009). Safety leaders should consider peer influence as one important factor in the use of PPE as well as interventions such as training, adequate PPE supply, and positive reinforcement as a package.

In another example of the impact of safety culture, Lowe (2008) surveyed 5,131 allied healthcare personnel, including emergency medical staff, community health personnel, and long-term care providers, about safety culture. Lowe reported that in the healthcare setting, teamwork, fair workplace processes, supportive and people-centered supervisors, leadership, a learning environment, and evidence that employers were working collaboratively to improve the work environment contributed to a culture that values safety. This broader research base that examines safety culture influences and barriers should be further explored in order to inform the work of healthcare organizations.

An in-depth review of Canada's experience with severe acute respiratory syndrome (SARS) by the SARS Commission emphasized the importance of a robust safety culture in healthcare facilities and pointed to the need for close cooperation between infection control and occupational safety and health programs and personnel (Possamai, 2007). Although safety culture issues in health care go well beyond a discussion of PPE, they are important components of those discussions. Recent research on organizational factors that impact the use of PPE (Cavazza and Serpe, 2009; Lombardi et al., 2009; Olson et al., 2009) has reinforced many of the factors identified in the 2008 IOM report, including

- availability of and participation in training and refresher courses,
- supervisor use of PPE,
- peer use of PPE,
- organizational support for worker safety and health—the extent to which the company minimizes hazards and prioritizes safety goals. Support is also evidenced by senior manager support of

safety practices and the level of encouragement for worker participation in health and safety discussions,

- positive reinforcement of individual compliance behavior, and
- negative reinforcement (e.g., verbal warnings).

Nichol and colleagues (2008) reported results from 177 nurses in 2 acute care hospitals in Canada. They found that compliance with PPE use was significantly related to organizational support for health and safety (however, no details were provided on what constituted organizational support). Other factors positively affecting the use of facial PPE included full-time employment status, more than 5 years of experience as a nurse, monthly or more frequent use of PPE, and belief in media coverage about the risks of communicable diseases. The absence of job hindrances, such as heavy workloads, was an important contributor.

Saint and colleagues (2009) conducted telephone and in-person interviews with 86 hospital staff in 14 U.S. hospitals about barriers to implementing evidence-based practices to prevent healthcare-associated infections. The authors identified two types of personnel barriers: "active resisters" and "organizational constipators." Active resisters were identified as hospital staff who actively and openly opposed changes in practice. One person identified this group as "entrenched culture." Another type of active resister was one who had competing authorities on new practice implementation, such as hospital policy being in conflict with Centers for Disease Control and Prevention guidelines. Organizational constipators tended to be mid- to high-level executives who prevented or delayed certain actions, thereby acting as barriers to evidence-based change implementation. They appeared to undercut changes and put their own interests ahead of those of organizations and patients. Strategies to overcome these behaviors need to be identified and implemented.

Additional studies point to the need for better training, equipment, and facilities. Ganczak and Szych (2007) conducted research on 601 surgical nurses in Poland and found that compliance with PPE varied considerably, ranging from 83 percent compliance with glove use to only 9 percent compliance with eye protection. Only 5 percent routinely used PPE when in contact with potentially infectious material. Compliance was higher among nurses who had received training in infection control. The most common reason reported for noncompliance was lack of PPE availability (37 percent). These findings related to adequate training were also found in a survey of 1,290 healthcare personnel as demonstrating the organization's commitment to keeping employees informed and up to date on best practices (Yassi et al., 2007). Yassi and colleagues (2009) used questionnaires, workplace assessments, and discussion groups at a South African hospital to gather information from health and safety representatives and occupational health practitioners. Findings showed weaknesses in knowing how to use N95 respirators and handle sharps, as well as limited supplies and training related to practice procedures. Turnberg and investigators (2008) conducted a survey of 653 hospital staff in 5 medical centers in Washington state and found lack of knowledge by healthcare personnel about, and limited training on, recommended infection control practices and PPE usage, as well as limited resource support. Investigators indicate there is a clear need to identify and reduce barriers to safe practice.

Recent research highlights the importance of the worker–task interface and work organization factors. Previous PPE research has often shown that physicians display poorer compliance than other categories of healthcare personnel. Although some recent data confirm this gradation (Manian and Ponzillo, 2007), other work suggests that these differences may be at least partially related to task assignments and the general organization of work (Chiang et al., 2008). Chiang and colleagues found that physicians complied better than nurses with PPE requirements during resuscitation activities in an intensive care unit. In this study, the poorer compliance of nurses was linked to the lack of specific task assignments, inadequate preparation for procedures, and the spatial characteristics and arrangement of the workspace. Lack of readily available PPE and time pressures continue to play a role in poor compliance (Shigayeva et al., 2007; Visentin et al., 2009). Other research shows that compliance may be more problematic in healthcare settings where staff vary on a day-to-day basis or rotate in and out of the setting (Trick et al., 2007). Job and task design, workgroup factors, supervisory practices, and other micro- and macro-work organization factors may also help to explain observed inconsistencies in compliance rates among healthcare personnel. These inconsistencies have been attributed previously to individual characteristics, such as job category, training level, job tenure, age, and even gender.

Individual Factors

Research published since 2007 on healthcare personnel and PPE shows that a number of individual factors continue to contribute to poor compliance and other safety-related outcomes. Three sets of factors deserve mention. First, studies continue to show knowledge gaps and training deficiencies among healthcare personnel with respect to proper PPE usage, modes of transmission, and other infection control topics. Research by Bryce and colleagues (2008) found that even though healthcare personnel may use appropriate PPE, they often do so incorrectly or incompletely. Examples include not doing a fit check after donning a respirator, continuing to use familiar devices regardless of fit test results, and not getting fit tested annually. Composite compliance and comfort scores were assessed for use of N95 respirators and eye protection (goggles, face shields, and other protective eyewear) among nurses, respiratory therapists, and other healthcare personnel at a tertiary care hospital that provides treatment for patients infected with tuberculosis (Bryce et al., 2008). For respirators, the composite compliance score was 86 percent of full compliance, and eye protection use was 74 percent of full compliance. No significant differences in compliance were observed for the three different models of N95 respirators used. The composite comfort score for N95 respirators was 68 percent of full comfort. For protective eyewear, the ability to see clearly was significantly and positively associated with both compliance and comfort. No association was reported between compliance and comfort for either respirators or protective eyewear. Healthcare personnel reported that they "felt better protected" with N95 respirators than with face masks.

Knowledge gaps also have been identified with respect to properly removing PPE (Hitoto et al., 2009), differentiating the protection levels offered by different types of PPE and PPE materials (Kanjirath et al., 2009), and having familiarity with newer protective devices (Ellison et al., 2007). This research highlights the fact that most PPE compliance behaviors are not simple, discrete actions. Rather, they are sets or sequences of behaviors that can vary under different circumstances. Total and perfect compliance with PPE use is a daunting task under the best of circumstances.

Second, research continues to indicate that healthcare personnel often rely on their own personal assessments of risk in deciding whether or not to use PPE. Results from a study by Visentin and colleagues (2009) suggest that, despite administrative directives, emergency medical technicians may fail to use certain PPE when they are not convinced it is needed in particular situations. Shigayeva and colleagues (2007) produced similar findings with respect to barrier protection during the SARS outbreak in Canada. One study found that healthcare personnel may believe they know more about PPE and infection control than they actually do (Shigayeva et al., 2007). Studies on the willingness of healthcare providers to work during crises involving infectious diseases have shown that having an adequate supply of PPE is an influential factor in being willing to respond and work (Balicer et al., 2010; Chaffee, 2009; Gershon et al., 2010a; Mackler et al., 2007; Wicker et al., 2009).

Third, recent research shows that healthcare personnel still believe that PPE can interfere with the patient–provider relationship and/or reduce the quality of care. For example, concerns about PPE include decreases in the field of vision or reductions in manual dexterity (Daugherty et al., 2009; Ellison et al., 2007; Visentin et al., 2009). Fifty-four healthcare personnel in a hospital emergency department were asked to wear a respirator (P2, an N95 equivalent) for a 4-week period during the influenza season whenever they were working within 1 meter of a patient with respiratory symptoms (Seale et al., 2009). During the first week, 24.1 percent of the participants wore the respirator "occasionally," while 42.6 percent never wore the respirator. In week 2, only 3 of the 54 participants wore the respirator "on most shifts." During weeks 3 and 4, only 1 healthcare worker wore the respirator "on most shifts." By week 4, 70.4 percent of the healthcare personnel reported that they never wore the respirator. Their reasons were that it was hot, was difficult to breathe through, interfered with patient communication, and had to be stored somewhere between uses.

Patient perceptions of PPE and its impact on provider behaviors is an area of ongoing research. Recent findings are providing insights into patient expectations and preferences with respect to PPE. Routine use of PPE by dental care providers seems to be well accepted by patients and expected as the norm (Molinari, 2010). Using a set of pictures of physicians with transparent face shields and traditional surgical masks, Forgie and colleagues (2009) asked parents and children (ages 4 to 10) which set of physicians they would prefer for patient care. Although 62 percent of parents thought their children would choose face shields, 59 percent of the children did not have a preference and found neither set to be frightening. A survey of dental patients found that face mask use was preferred by a majority of the patients (72 percent), with younger patients (< 46 years of age) more supportive of face mask use (McKenna et al., 2007).

Interventions to Improve Infection Control
and/or PPE Compliance

Gammon and colleagues (2007) conducted a literature review of research on healthcare worker compliance with standard/universal infection control precautions. They found suboptimal compliance in 24 studies that assessed compliance and only short-term improvements in the 13 studies examining interventions (primarily training classes) to improve compliance. In most intervention studies, compliance was monitored for only a few months after the intervention, and compliance often returned to baseline levels within a relatively short time. For example, a study of emergency medical services personnel found poor retention of donning and doffing procedures at a point approximately 6 months after the initial training (Northington et al., 2007).

Since 2007, several training-related intervention studies have been done. Howard and colleagues (2009) tested a clean-practice protocol and found that it significantly improved hand decontamination and overall infection control after 3 months. However, this was a small study without a control or comparison group. No further follow-up assessment was conducted to assess long-term maintenance.

Hon and colleagues (2008) reported that an online infection control course adequately transferred knowledge regarding PPE selection and use. But again, no control group was used, and the online course was not compared to other instructional modalities. In one better designed study, Trick and colleagues (2007) conducted a 3-year intervention study of hand hygiene and glove usage. Hygiene significantly improved in two of the three treatment hospitals compared with the control hospital. The best performing hospital also showed a reduced incidence of antimicrobial-resistant bacteria infections. The third treatment hospital showed insignificant improvement. This hospital was a large, public teaching hospital. These recent studies tentatively suggest that multicomponent training interventions may be more effective than single-component efforts and that communications and convenient reminders placed throughout the work environment may boost compliance. Training and other interventions that make use of social-cognitive and other behavioral theories also appear to hold promise (Godin et al., 2008).

Use of PPE by Home and Community
Healthcare Personnel

A segment of the healthcare workforce often overlooked in discussions on PPE and pandemic influenza planning is the more than 1.5 million home healthcare personnel and those working in community settings other than hospitals and large clinics (e.g., schools, physician's offices, long-term care settings) in the United States (Baron et al., 2009). These settings do not generally offer the administrative and environmental safety controls that should be available in hospitals or other large healthcare facilities. A recent study examined factors relevant to the willingness and ability of home healthcare personnel to take care of their patients during an influenza pandemic (Gershon et al., 2010b). Of the 384 home healthcare personnel responding to the questionnaire, 16 percent (57 workers) reported that their employer gave them a "respirator mask," with 41 workers reporting that they received training on how to use the equipment and 16 reporting that they had been fit tested on the equipment they were provided. When asked about whether they would be willing to provide care during a pandemic to their current patients, respiratory protection was a significant factor, with willingness to work being associated with "being confident that the mask would protect me" (51 percent) and "being given a respirator mask" (47 percent).

Hinkin and colleagues (2008) conducted a literature review and found poor compliance with standard precautions among community nurses. Employers must provide suitable facilities, sufficient supplies of PPE, and adequate training. The authors note that most research has been done in hospitals, which has only limited applicability to other community settings.

SUMMARY OF PROGRESS

Research during the past several years reveals modest gains in understanding that self-protective behavior in the healthcare settings involves a constellation of interacting and independent components. At a minimum, consideration should be given to the user, the device, the task, and the general work and organizational context. Daugherty and colleagues (2009) found that knowledge and task hindrances were related to poor compliance among critical care clinicians, with the authors concluding that organizational factors were more important than individual factors in explaining PPE usage. The growing acknowledgment of contextual and organizational factors means that research on PPE and healthcare personnel is closing in on the larger body of occupational safety research, which increasingly emphasizes contextual and organizational factors in understanding occupational safety performance.

Although there are clear gaps and deficiencies in our knowledge base about PPE usage in health care, existing knowledge is sufficient to recommend a four-pronged strategy for immediate implementation. The four elements are as follows: (1) deliberate planning and preparation at the leadership and organizational levels; (2) comprehensive training, including supervisors and managers; (3) widespread and convenient availability of appropriate PPE devices; and (4) accountability at all levels of the organization. In essence, there should be universal acknowledgment that PPE usage is an integral component of providing quality health care. As with other priorities, this aspect of healthcare delivery needs to be planned carefully at the organizational/institutional level, managers and frontline workers alike need to understand and accept their roles and responsibilities, and PPE usage needs to be as easy and convenient as possible. PPE should be factored into all decisions involving task design, staffing, and work assignments. Input from frontline workers should be used to facilitate planning and decision making and maximize acceptance. Environmental/engineering controls should be utilized wherever possible to control exposures, with PPE used as a supplement or alternative when environmental/engineering controls are not sufficient or feasible. The overall implementation of the PPE program should be monitored regularly, with the goals of continuous improvement, adoption of best practices, and accountability of both supervisor and worker.

FINDINGS AND RESEARCH NEEDS

This is an opportune time for research on promoting and enhancing healthcare worker safety and the use of PPE. As noted throughout the chapter, extensive work has been done in recent years on improving patient safety. Efforts are needed to build on those efforts and identify the linkages between patient safety and worker safety, particularly with the use of PPE. Additionally, safety research conducted in other types of work settings has potential applicability to improving safety performance and PPE use in health care. Furthermore, much can be learned from recent experience by healthcare personnel and organizations during the

2009 H1N1 influenza, and exploring lessons learned can be instructive for moving research efforts forward. Increased knowledge and communication on the severity of the disease will also be important as decisions are made by organizations regarding PPE compliance. Box 4-1 highlights the committee's findings in this area.

The committee has identified the following research needs and recommendations. Some of these can and need to be addressed expeditiously; others will require longer-term efforts. The goals will be to identify and evaluate strategies to mitigate organizational and other barriers that limit the use of PPE by healthcare personnel and to identify incentives and enforcement mechanisms to ensure ongoing organizational commitment and continuous improvement. Efforts should be aimed across the spectrum of healthcare personnel and should consider language, educational, and cultural issues.

Studies have examined barriers to PPE use; however, research gaps remain on identifying effective strategies for sustaining PPE use related to training, policies, and actions, including assessment of the knowledge, attitudes, and priorities of healthcare personnel and senior management about PPE. Research is needed on the following issues:

- **PPE issues in health science school curriculums:** Studies are needed to determine the level of inclusion of contemporary concepts and applications regarding PPE in the curriculums of

---

BOX 4-1
Findings

- Self-protective behavior in healthcare settings involves a constellation of interacting and independent factors.
- Organizational and individual changes are complex, time consuming, and difficult to sustain.
- Personal protective equipment usage presents varied challenges across different types of healthcare settings.
- Existing knowledge is sufficient to begin to incorporate the following practices into PPE usage in health care: deliberate planning and preparation at the leadership and organizational levels; comprehensive training, including supervisors and managers; widespread and convenient availability of appropriate PPE devices; and accountability at all levels of the organization.

---

health science and allied health schools. These studies should include all levels of education where practice is a component. Recommendations should be made for closing identified gaps and improving the development, content, and dissemination of PPE training materials.

- **Healthcare worker safety culture:** Recent efforts focused on patient safety should be expanded to examine the worker safety climate specific to the healthcare arena and PPE use. This includes examining the applicability to health care of research findings in the areas of patient safety, high-reliability organizations, high-hazard industries, and general industry. Lessons learned from the experience with 2009 H1N1 influenza could be informative in identifying best practices, learning from organizations successful with PPE compliance by healthcare personnel as well as from those with lower rates of compliance, and examining issues relevant to PPE policy and implementation relevant to both large and small healthcare employers. To improve appropriate use of PPE, it will be vital to better understand the motivations and risk assessment processes used by healthcare personnel regarding use of and demand for PPE.
- **Incentives and enforcement:** Innovative approaches to incident reporting systems and other incentive and enforcement actions need to be examined that promote PPE use by fostering a strong and positive culture of safety in the workplace and learning from mistakes.
- **Task and work organization:** Efforts are needed to examine the contribution of task and work organization factors (how work processes are structured and managed) to PPE usage and other safe work practices in healthcare settings.
- **Metrics:** Similar to measures of the patient safety culture, metrics are needed to measure worker and organizational safety culture and use of PPE.
- **Varying healthcare settings:** In order to determine practice needs in different work settings, research is needed to examine and differentiate PPE policy and implementation strategies in large and small healthcare delivery settings.

RECOMMENDATIONS

Recommendation: <u>Explore Healthcare Safety Culture and Work Organization</u>
The National Institute for Occupational Safety and Health (NIOSH) and other relevant agencies, such as the Agency for Healthcare Research and Quality, and professional organizations should conduct research to better understand the role of safety culture and other behavioral and organizational factors on PPE usage in healthcare settings. These efforts should include

- conducting human factors and ergonomics research relevant to the design and organization of healthcare work tasks to improve worker safety by reducing hazardous exposures and effectively using PPE (e.g., reduce unnecessary PPE donning and doffing),
- exploring the links between patient safety and healthcare worker safety and health that are relevant to the use of PPE, and
- identifying and evaluating strategies to mitigate organizational barriers that limit the use of PPE by healthcare personnel.

Recommendation: <u>Identify and Disseminate Effective Leadership and Training Strategies and Other Interventions to Improve PPE Use</u>
NIOSH and other relevant agencies and professional organizations should support intervention effectiveness research to assess strategies, including innovative participatory approaches to training, for healthcare and supervisory staff at all levels to improve PPE usage and other related outcomes across the range of healthcare settings. To identify best practices, efforts should be made to

- conduct observational studies of PPE usage by healthcare personnel in different types of work settings;
- develop, implement, and evaluate comprehensive leadership and training strategies and interventions that go beyond simple knowledge-based training;

- design training interventions specifically for supervisory and managerial personnel in different types of healthcare settings;
- examine long-term practice change and safety culture implementation related to educational interventions;
- improve use and understanding of PPE by home and community healthcare personnel;
- develop assessment tools and metrics that take a broader approach to PPE and acknowledge the interaction of worker, task, and environmental factors; and
- be informed by a lessons-learned summit on PPE use by healthcare personnel during the 2009 H1N1 experience.

REFERENCES

Balicer, R. D., D. J. Barnett, C. B. Thompson, E. B. Hsu, C. L. Catlett, C. M. Watson, N. L. Semon, H. S. Gwon, and J. M. Links. 2010. Characterizing hospital workers' willingness to report to duty in an influenza pandemic through threat- and efficacy-based assessment. *BMC Public Health* 10:436.

Baron, S., K. McPhaul, S. Phillips, R. Gershon, and J. Lipscomb. 2009. Protecting home health care workers: A challenge to pandemic influenza preparedness planning. *American Journal of Public Health* 99(Suppl. 2):S301-S307.

Bryce, E., L. Forrester, S. Scharf, and M. Eshghpour. 2008. What do healthcare workers think? A survey of facial protection equipment user preferences. *Journal of Hospital Infection* 68(3):241-247.

Cavazza, N., and A. Serpe. 2009. Effects of safety climate on safety norm violations: Exploring the mediating role of attitudinal ambivalence toward personal protective equipment. *Journal of Safety Research* 40(4):277-283.

Chaffee, M. 2009. Willingness of health care personnel to work in a disaster: An integrative review of the literature. *Disaster Medicine and Public Health Preparedness* 3(1):42-56.

Chiang, W.-C., H.-C. Wang, S.-Y. Chen, L.-M. Chen, Y.-C. Yao, G. H.-M. Wu, P. C.-I. Ko, C.-W. Yang, M.-T. Tsai, C.-C. Hsai, C.-P. Su, S.-C. Chen, and M. H.-M. Ma. 2008. Lack of compliance with basic infection control measures during cardiopulmonary resuscitation—are we ready for another epidemic? *Resuscitation* 77(3):356-362.

Daugherty, E. L., T. M. Perl, D. M. Needham, L. Rubinson, A. Bilderback, and C. S. Rand. 2009. The use of personal protective equipment for control of influenza among critical care clinicians: A survey study. *Critical Care Medicine* 37(4):1210-1216.

Ellison, A. M., M. Kotelchuck, and H. Bauchner. 2007. Standard precautions in the pediatric emergency department: Knowledge, attitudes, and behaviors of pediatric and emergency medicine residents. *Pediatric Emergency Care* 23(12):877-880.

Forgie, S. E., J. Reitsma, D. Spady, B. Wright, and K. Stobart. 2009. The "fear factor" for surgical masks and face shields, as perceived by children and their parents. *Pediatrics* 124(4):e777-e781.

Gaba, D. M., S. J. Singer, A. D. Sinaiko, J. D. Bowen, and A. P. Ciavarelli. 2003. Differences in safety climate between hospital personnel and naval aviators. *Human Factors: The Journal of the Human Factors and Ergonomics Society* 45(2):173-185.

Gammon, J., H. Morgan-Samuel, and D. Gould. 2007. A review of the evidence for suboptimal compliance of healthcare practitioners to standard/universal infection control precautions. *Journal of Clinical Nursing* 17(2):157-167.

Ganczak, M., and Z. Szych. 2007. Surgical nurses and compliance with personal protective equipment. *Journal of Hospital Infection* 66(4):346-351.

Gershon, R. R. M., D. Vlahov, S. A. Felknor, D. Vesley, P. C. Johnson, G. L. Delcios, and L. R. Murphy. 1995. Compliance with universal precautions among health care workers at three regional hospitals. *American Journal of Infection Control* 23(4):225-236.

Gershon, R. R., L. A. Magda, K. A. Qureshi, H. E. Riley, E. Scanlon, M. T. Carney, R. J. Richards, and M. F. Sherman. 2010a. Factors associated with the ability and willingness of essential workers to report to duty during a pandemic. *Journal of Occupational and Environmental Medicine* 52(10):995-1003.

Gershon, R. R. M., L. A. Magda, A. N. Canton, H. E. M. Riley, F. Wiggins, W. Young, and M. F. Sherman. 2010b. Pandemic-related ability and willingness in home healthcare workers. *American Journal of Disaster Medicine* 5(1):15-26.

Godin, G., A. Belanger-Gravel, M. Eccles, and J. Grimshaw. 2008. Healthcare professionals' intentions and behaviours: A systematic review of studies based on social cognitive theories. *Implementation Science* 3:36.

Hinkin, J., J. Gammon, and J. Cutter. 2008. Review of personal protection equipment used in practice. *British Journal of Community Nursing* 13(1):14-19.

Hitoto, H., A. Kouatchet, L. Dube, C. Lemarie, A. Mercat, M. L. Joly-Guillou, and M. Eveillard. 2009. Factors affecting compliance with glove removal after contact with a patient or environment in four intensive care units. *Journal of Hospital Infection* 71(2):186-188.

Hofmann, D. A., R. Jacobs, and F. Landy. 1995. High reliability process industries: Individual, micro, and macro organizational influences on safety performance. *Journal of Safety Research* 26(3):131-149.

Hon, C. Y., B. Gamage, E. A. Bryce, J. LoChang, A. Yassi, D. Maultsaid, and S. Yu. 2008. Personal protective equipment in health care: Can online infection control courses transfer knowledge and improve proper selection and use? *American Journal of Infection Control* 36(10):e33-e37.

Howard, D. P., C. Williams, S. Sen, A. Shah, J. Daurka, R. Bird, A. Loh, and A. Howard. 2009. A simple effective clean practice protocol significantly improves hand decontamination and infection control measures in the acute surgical setting. *Infection* 37(1):34-38.

IOM (Institute of Medicine). 2000. *To err is human: Building a safer health system*. Washington, DC: National Academy Press.

———. 2008. *Preparing for an influenza pandemic: Personal protective equipment for healthcare workers*. Washington, DC: The National Academies Press.

Kanjirath, P. P., A. E. Coplen, J. C. Chapman, M. C. Peters, and M. R. Inglehart. 2009. Effectiveness of gloves and infection control in dentistry: Student and provider perspectives. *Journal of Dental Education* 73(5):571-580.

Lombardi, D. A., S. K. Verma, M. J. Brennan, and M. J. Perry. 2009. Factors influencing worker use of personal protective eyewear. *Accident Analysis and Prevention* 41(4):755-762.

Lowe, G. S. 2008. The role of healthcare work environments in shaping a safety culture. *Healthcare Quarterly* 11(2):42-51.

Mackler, N., W. Wilkerson, and S. Cinti. 2007. Will first-responders show up for work during a pandemic? Lessons from a smallpox vaccination survey of paramedics. *Disaster Management and Response* 5(2):45-48.

Manian, F. A., and J. J. Ponzillo. 2007. Compliance with routine use of gowns by healthcare workers (HCWs) and non-HCW visitors on entry into the rooms of patients under contact precautions. *Infection Control and Hospital Epidemiology* 28(3):337-340.

McKenna, G., G. R. Lillywhite, and N. Maini. 2007. Patient preferences for dental clinical attire: A cross-sectional survey in a dental hospital. *British Dental Journal* 203(12):681-685.

Molinari, J. 2010, June 3. *Dental community experience*. PowerPoint presented at the IOM Workshop on Current Research Issues—Personal Protective Equipment for Healthcare Workers to Prevent Transmission of Pandemic Influenza and Other Viral Respiratory Infections, Washington, DC. http://iom.edu/~/media/Files/Activity%20Files/PublicHealth/PPECurrentResearch/2010-JUN-3/Molinari%20-%20Panel%204.pdf (accessed March 14, 2011).

Nichol, K., P. Bigelow, L. O'Brien-Pallas, A. McGeer, M. Manno, and D. L. Holness. 2008. The individual, environmental, and organizational factors that influence nurses' use of facial protection to prevent occupational transmission of communicable respiratory illness in acute care hospitals. *American Journal of Infection Control* 36(7):481-487.

Northington, W. E., G. M. Mahoney, M. E. Hahn, J. Suyama, and D. Hostler. 2007. Training retention of level C personal protective equipment use by emergency medical services personnel. *Academic Emergency Medicine* 14(10):846-849.

Olson, R., A. Grosshuesch, S. Schmidt, M. Gray, and B. Wipfli. 2009. Observational learning and workplace safety: The effects of viewing the collective behavior of multiple social models on the use of personal protective equipment. *Journal of Safety Research* 40(5):383-387.

Possamai, M. A. 2007. SARS and health worker safety: Lessons for influenza pandemic planning and response. *HealthcarePapers* 8(1):18-28.

Roberts, K. H. 1990. Some characteristics of one type of high reliability organization. *Organization Science* 1(2):160-176.

Rochlin, G. I. 1999. Safe operation as a social construct. *Ergonomics* 42(11):1549-1560.

Saint, S., C. P. Kowalski, J. Banaszak-Holl, J. Forman, L. Damschroder, and S. L. Krein. 2009. How active resisters and organizational constipators affect health care-acquired infection prevention efforts. *Joint Commission Journal on Quality and Patient Safety* 35(5):239-246.

Seale, H., S. Corbett, D. E. Dwyer, and C. R. MacIntyre. 2009. Feasibility exercise to evaluate the use of particulate respirators by emergency department staff during the 2007 influenza season. *Infection Control and Hospital Epidemiology* 30(7):710-712.

Shigayeva, A., K. Green, J. M. Raboud, B. Henry, A. E. Simor, M. Vearncombe, D. Zoutman, M. Loeb, and A. McGeer. 2007. Factors associated with critical-care healthcare workers' adherence to recommended barrier precautions during the Toronto severe acute respiratory syndrome outbreak. *Infection Control and Hospital Epidemiology* 28(11):1275-1283.

Singer, S. J., D. M. Gaba, J. J. Geppert, A. D. Sinaiko, S. K. Howard, and K. C. Park. 2003. The culture of safety: Results of an organization-wide survey in 15 california hospitals. *Quality and Safety in Health Care* 12(2):112-118.

Singer, S., S. Lin, A. Falwell, D. Gaba, and L. Baker. 2009. Relationship of safety climate and safety performance in hospitals. *Health Services Research* 44(2p1):399-421.

Trick, W. E., M. O. Vernon, S. F. Welbel, P. Demarais, M. K. Hayden, and R. A. Weinstein. 2007. Multicenter intervention program to increase adherence to hand hygiene recommendations and glove use and to reduce the incidence of antimicrobial resistance. *Infection Control and Hospital Epidemiology* 28(1):42-49.

Tucker, A. L., S. J. Singer, J. E. Hayes, and A. Falwell. 2008. Front-line staff perspectives on opportunities for improving the safety and efficiency of hospital work systems. *Health Services Research* 43(5p2):1807-1829.

Turnberg, W., W. Daniell, N. Seixas, T. Simpson, J. Van Buren, E. Lipkin, and J. Duchin. 2008. Appraisal of recommended respiratory infection control practices in primary care and emergency department settings. *American Journal of Infection Control* 36(4):268-275.

Visentin, L. M., S. J. Bondy, B. Schwartz, and L. J. Morrison. 2009. Use of personal protective equipment during infectious disease outbreak and nonoutbreak conditions: A survey of emergency medical technicians. *Canadian Journal of Emergency Medicine* 11(1):44-56.

Weick, K. E., K. M. Sutcliffe, and D. Obstfeld. 1999. Organizing for high reliability: Processes of collective mindfulness. In *Research in organizational behavior.* Vol. 1, edited by B. M. Staw and R. I. Sutton. Stanford, CA: Elsevier Science/JAI Press. Pp. 81-123.

Wicker, S., H. F. Rabenau, and R. Gottschalk. 2009. [Influenza pandemic: Would healthcare workers come to work? An analysis of the ability and willingness to report to duty]. *Bundesgesundheitsblatt Gesundheitsforschung Gesundheitsschutz* 52(8):862-869.

Yassi, A., K. Lockhart, R. Copes, M. Kerr, M. Corbiere, E. Bryce, Q. Danyluk, D. Keen, S. Yu, C. Kidd, M. Fitzgerald, R. Thiessen, B. Gamage, D. Patrick, P. Bigelow, and S. Saunders. 2007. Determinants of healthcare workers' compliance with infection control procedures. *Healthcare Quarterly* 10(1):44-52.

Yassi, A., L. E. Nophale, L. Dybka, E. Bryce, W. Kruger, and J. Spiegel. 2009. Building capacity to secure healthier and safer working conditions for healthcare workers: A South African-Canadian collaboration. *International Journal of Occupational and Environmental Health* 15(4):360-369.

5

Policy Research and Implementation: Healthcare Systems, Standards, and Certification

The emergence of 2009 H1N1 influenza and the ensuing dilemmas regarding personal protective equipment (PPE) for healthcare personnel highlighted challenges in healthcare delivery policy at institutional, state, regional, and national levels as well as policies about the relevant standards and certification processes. This chapter highlights issues regarding standards and policies for PPE for healthcare personnel and summarizes the experience and literature on the 2009 H1N1 pandemic relevant to PPE. The chapter also provides the committee's recommendations on the next policy and regulatory steps needed to address the current challenges and improve PPE for healthcare personnel.

PPE STANDARDS AND CERTIFICATION

As described in Chapter 1 (with more detail provided in Box 5-1), a number of state and federal agencies and organizations have regulatory, standards-setting, and policy responsibilities regarding PPE for healthcare personnel. This section highlights several recent and ongoing efforts with potential impact on PPE for healthcare personnel, some of which require further attention and action.

Recent and Ongoing Changes to Standards and Regulations

Two recent regulatory changes implemented by the Occupational Safety and Health Administration (OSHA) impact workplace access to

PPE and voluntary consensus standards. A Final Rule, issued in November 2007, requires employers to provide PPE at no cost to their employees; this change took the burden of responsibility off the employees, who in some cases had been paying for their own protective equipment (29 Code of Federal Regulations [CFR] 1910.132; OSHA, 2007). In September 2009, a Final Rule was promulgated to address various revisions of the voluntary consensus standards as they applied to several types of PPE, including eye and face protection (29 CFR 1910.133), head protection (29 CFR 1910.135), and foot protection (29 CFR 1910.136; OSHA, 2009). Because many consensus standards are updated on a regular basis, the new OSHA regulations state that the employer needs to supply PPE that meets the current voluntary consensus standard or either of the past two versions of that standard; thus employers do not have to purchase new PPE every time a consensus standard is revised.

In October 2009, the National Institute for Occupational Safety and Health (NIOSH) proposed total inward leakage (TIL) requirements for the certification of negative-pressure, tight-fitting respirators. The new regulation would require that half-facepiece, air-purifying respirators (including filtering facepiece respirators such as the N95 respirator) be fit tested to an anthropometrically selected panel of wearers. Respirators would need to be able to achieve an acceptable fit to a wide range of faces. Two public meetings have been held, and the docket for public comments closed in September 2010 (NIOSH, 2010a). NIOSH will evaluate the comments received and may then release a final standard. The goal is to improve the fit of respirators.

In 2009, California became the first state in the nation to issue a standard requiring employers to protect healthcare personnel from influenza and other viral respiratory diseases when it promulgated its aerosol-transmissible diseases standard (California Code of Regulations, 2010). This standard uses Centers for Disease Control and Prevention (CDC) guidelines and terminology to classify whether an aerosol-transmissible disease requires droplet precautions (use of face masks is permitted) or requires aerosol precautions (respiratory protection is required using N95s at a minimum, and where aerosol-generating procedures are performed, a powered air-purifying respirator [PAPR] or greater level of protection is required) (Siegel et al., 2007). Thus, by adopting the CDC guidelines, healthcare employers in California would, for example, protect personnel against seasonal influenza using face masks, while exposures to measles virus would require respirators (N95s or greater). For novel or unknown pathogens (e.g., the 2009 H1N1 pandemic influenza virus), the California standard sets the default protection level at airborne precautions where use of respirators would be required (California Code of Regulations, 2010).

Recent efforts have also focused on voluntary consensus standards development and on third-party conformity assessment. ASTM International announced in April 2010 the establishment of a working group that will develop test methods to assess the effectiveness of antimicrobial gloves (ASTM International, 2010a). Additionally, a task group within the subcommittee on consumer rubber products has begun developing standards that focus on preventing the transfer of microorganisms through the use of antimicrobial agents (ASTM International, 2010c). Furthermore, an ASTM International subcommittee is focused on developing a product certification process for protective clothing and equipment that would include an option for third-party independent verification that the product met the relevant performance standards (ASTM International, 2010b).

BOX 5-1
Existing Standards, Guidelines, and Certification Processes

Food and Drug Administration (FDA)
    Medical device legislation beginning in 1937 and amended in 1976 makes the FDA the principal agency for clearing personal protective equipment (PPE) for use by healthcare personnel. PPE devices used in healthcare environments are considered medical devices and are regulated as either Class I or Class II devices. Class I devices are considered low risk to the user, and the basic requirement is that the manufacturer meet general standards for good manufacturing processes. Some Class I devices require that the manufacturer provide a 510(k) submission and demonstrate that the device meets specific voluntary standards and is substantively equivalent to a similar "predicate" device currently on the market. Examples of Class I devices that require a 510(k) submission include surgeon and examination gloves. Class II devices are considered intermediate risk and must be cleared through the 510(k) process before they are allowed to be marketed. Surgical gowns, face masks, and respirators are also categorized as Class II devices.
    The FDA does not conduct tests on medical devices; the agency reviews data submitted by manufacturers to demonstrate that the product has been tested (by the manufacturer or an independent testing organization) to meet specified consensus standards. Respirators are required to be certified by the National Institute for Occupational Safety and Health (NIOSH) and must meet additional requirements for flammability and fluid protection. The FDA does not have any specific PPE requirements for protection against infectious diseases such as influenza. Therefore, masks and respirators have requirements that are

continued

specifically geared for surgical room use, not for protection against influenza or other viral respiratory diseases. The FDA has begun clearing such devices that make claims for antiviral protection.

FDA regulations are designed to control the manufacture and sale of PPE. These regulations do not specifically apply to employers or employees. Requirements regarding the use of PPE in the healthcare workplace are overseen by the Occupational Safety and Health Administration (OSHA), along with state and local agencies and employers.

National Institute for Occupational Safety and Health

NIOSH is the principal governmental agency with responsibility for testing and certifying respirators. The National Personal Protective Technology Laboratory (NPPTL) establishes the testing requirements and performs tests on respirators submitted by manufacturers. Testing and certification requirements are incorporated in the Code of Federal Regulations (42 CFR Part 84). Once a respirator is certified, the manufacturer is not required to resubmit the device for further testing unless modifications are made.

NIOSH respirator testing and certification requirements are specific to the type of respirator (e.g., air-purifying, self-contained breathing apparatus) and are not specific to the type of workplace where they will be used. There is no specific certification of respirators for healthcare personnel or for protection against infectious agents such as influenza. However, as discussed in Chapter 3, NPPTL staff and other researchers have studied the performance of certified filters against nanoparticles that would be applicable to virons and also have conducted some research with antiviral filters. The NIOSH certification process does not evaluate or indicate the efficacy of antiviral treatments that may be applied to filters on certified respirators.

NIOSH does not certify other forms of PPE, such as gloves and goggles, that would be relevant to the protection of healthcare personnel. NIOSH staff do participate in the development of voluntary consensus standards for other PPE and perform some research in these areas (IOM, 2010).

Occupational Safety and Health Administration

OSHA has the primary responsibility for enforcing the proper use of PPE in the workplace, including in healthcare facilities. The two main regulations relevant to PPE use by healthcare personnel relevant to viral respiratory diseases are 29 CFR 1910.134, which governs the use of respirators, and 29 CFR 1910.132, which governs the use of PPE other than respirators. All respirators used by healthcare personnel must be NIOSH certified, and their use must be part of a respiratory protection program that includes attention to issues regarding medical clearance, fit testing (where applicable), and training. OSHA requires that other types of PPE meet specified voluntary consensus standards (in some cases—e.g., for eye and face protection—OSHA regulations include additional specifications as noted in 29 CFR 1910.133). OSHA does not have specific standards covering the use of PPE by healthcare personnel and does not require that such PPE be cleared by the FDA.

Other Agencies and Organizations

A number of other organizations also impact the use of PPE by healthcare personnel. The Centers for Disease Control and Prevention (CDC) provides infection control guidance, including guidance on the use of respirators and masks by healthcare personnel for protection against influenza. During the 2009 H1N1 pandemic, the CDC infection control guidelines for healthcare personnel during seasonal influenza (which recommend droplet infection control precautions, e.g., a face mask for non-aerosol-generating procedures) were changed to recommend airborne precautions involving the use of respirators (respirators are recommended for aerosol-generating procedures in both). However, some state health agencies or local healthcare facilities continued to recommend face masks consistent with seasonal influenza guidelines for the use of respirators and masks. In summer 2010, the CDC guidelines were revised to reflect the seasonal infection control precautions based on availability of an effective vaccine and updated knowledge about the risk of hospitalization and death from 2009 H1N1 influenza (CDC, 2010).

The Joint Commission provides accreditation for many hospitals and a variety of other employers of healthcare personnel, such as home healthcare agencies. The use of PPE is included in the Joint Commission's requirements for employers.

State and local health agencies provide guidance and licensing to employers of healthcare personnel. These agencies provide assistance to employers in the case of pandemic influenza that may include stockpiling of PPE and offering guidance on what type of PPE is appropriate for specific tasks.

Standards development organizations (such as the American National Standards Institute and ASTM International) work through professional organizations and standards development committees to develop voluntary consensus standards that specify testing methods and performance expectations. Standards-development committees include experts who represent manufacturers, employers, users, and government regulators. Each standards-development organization has its own rules about the balance of these committees and voting. Most standards must be updated on a regular basis (e.g., 5 years) or they are withdrawn. Standards may specify whether PPE must be tested by an independent third party or whether the manufacturer can perform the testing.

Moving Forward on PPE Standards and Certification

Many of the issues that require activity by regulatory agencies for worker protection regarding PPE use during pandemic influenza involve respirators and masks. Face (eye), hand, and body protection issues all involve barriers, such as goggles or face shields, gloves, and gowns, which should provide an adequate barrier against influenza transmission provided that they cover the exposed area.

A major challenge in preventing influenza transmission continues to be clarifying the modes of transmission (Chapter 2). Occupational safety and health principles emphasize the importance of protecting the worker, particularly when dealing with hazards of unknown severity or health impacts. For novel respiratory viruses, the committee reiterates the statements in the 2008 Institute of Medicine report regarding transmission of influenza A: "[w]ithout knowing the contributions of each of the possible route(s) of transmission, all routes must be considered probable and consequential" (IOM, 2008, p. 53).

As reiterated throughout this report, PPE is one part of a comprehensive infection control program that includes engineering, administrative, and workplace controls, including vaccination. Because transmission of influenza occurs in the community and does not just occur in healthcare settings from patients and coworkers, vaccination—when effective—is a preventive measure that offers protection that is not tied to a specific workplace setting or on-the-job practices and equipment.

Face Masks and Face Shields

As discussed throughout this report, one of the most contentious issues regarding PPE to prevent influenza transmission is the use of masks versus respirators. Protection of healthcare personnel is paramount in these discussions. For employers, the issues to consider include purchase and training costs. As discussed in Chapter 3, more research is needed to determine the extent and nature of the protection that face masks and face shields can provide against viral respiratory disease transmission; a role in providing contact and droplet spray has been suggested but remains unclear. As information becomes available that clarifies the PPE role that face masks and face shields play in preventing transmission of viral respiratory diseases, voluntary consensus standards and certification processes will need to be developed, implemented, and refined so that healthcare personnel and other consumers will have information on the effectiveness of these products.

OSHA's respiratory protection standard (29 CFR 1910.134) includes requirements for the selection, use, and maintenance of respirators. Since face masks are not respirators, they are not covered by this standard. OSHA general PPE standard (29 CFR 1910.132) applies to face shields and face masks; however, specific performance standards or other design or performance criteria for these products are not included in this OSHA regulation. To move forward with this issue, OSHA could work with other agencies and organizations to identify relevant voluntary consensus standard requirements and consider if selection, maintenance, storage, and inspection requirements for face masks and face shields should be detailed in OSHA regulations to provide further protection for healthcare personnel.

Respirators

Fit and fit testing Several significant policy and regulatory issues exist regarding respirator fit and fit testing that could impact healthcare worker safety and health in the midst of an influenza pandemic or an outbreak of a novel viral respiratory disease. During an emergency situation, employers may run out of respirators that have been fit tested on personnel and may be unable to obtain additional supplies from the same manufacturer or an emergency stockpile. If supplies of other types of respirators are available, then OSHA requirements stipulate the need for repeat fit testing with the new type of respirator to ensure proper fit and protection (29 CFR 1910.134). The challenge during an emergency situation could be the need to do fit testing for large numbers of workers in a short period of time. Therefore, a user seal check or other quick method of determining the fit of a respirator needs to be developed and recommended by NIOSH and/or OSHA as a temporary measure to be used during emergencies until the required fit testing can be completed.

A second issue is that the current NIOSH respirator certification program has no requirement for a TIL test for filtering facepiece respirators (e.g., many N95 respirators). Therefore, a respirator may be NIOSH certified for filtration efficiency, but have poor-fitting characteristics and be unable to fit a large number of workers. When health agencies or employers stockpile respirators, they may choose devices based on cost and availability but may not have the knowledge about how well the device will fit their population. This issue became widely recognized during the 2009 H1N1 pandemic when a California stockpile of respirators was used and healthcare personnel could not obtain a satisfactory fit (NIOSH, 2010b). The proposed respirator TIL regulations would assist in addressing this issue and provide employers and workers with better fitting respirators.

PAPRs During an influenza pandemic, some healthcare personnel who do not normally wear respirators may need to wear them. These individuals are unlikely to be able to obtain a respirator fit test in a timely manner. In addition, some individuals may have facial hair or other facial features that do not allow them to be fitted adequately to a typical N95 or other tight-fitting respirator. These individuals would need to be assigned a loose-fitting PAPR. These types of respirators provide forced-flow filtered air but currently have high noise levels that are not conducive to healthcare tasks and patient interactions, including speech perception and listening to chest sounds. Efforts are underway by the National Personal Protective Technology Laboratory (NPPTL) to develop regulations for testing and approving lower flow PAPRs that would provide acceptable respiratory protection in a healthcare environment but emit less noise and thus be more useful for healthcare work that requires communication with patients. Expediting these efforts is critical to improving PPE for healthcare personnel.

Aerosol-transmissible disease standard   As noted above, California adopted an aerosol-transmissible diseases standard in 2009 (California Code of Regulations, 2010). The standard includes a list of diseases and pathogens that require airborne precautions as outlined by CDC, including "novel or unknown pathogens" (California Code of Regulations, 2010). The scope of airborne precaution measures includes the requirement for "at least the use of an N95 respirator" (Jensen et al., 2005). During the 2009 H1N1 pandemic, the California standard was the only workplace standard in the United States that required a mandatory level of worker protection to be provided to healthcare personnel. Other state and local health departments had access to the CDC and OSHA guidance, but practices at healthcare facilities varied in whether and when they followed airborne or droplet infection control precautions. In May 2010, OSHA issued a *Federal Register* notice requesting information on occupational exposure to infectious agents in health care and related settings (e.g., laboratories, medical examiner offices) (OSHA, 2010). OSHA needs to work toward the development of an aerosol-transmissible diseases standard that would provide adequate protection for healthcare personnel and that would, in situations of unknown or novel pathogens, default to providing full respiratory protection until more was known about the lethality or contagiousness of the disease.

Other regulatory issues   To gain approval for marketing as a medical device, the Food and Drug Administration (FDA) stipulates that the respirators must be NIOSH certified and meet flammability and fluid protection standards; these standards are not relevant for most situations in which workers must be protected from influenza. During the recent pandemic, the FDA identified non-cleared respirators that would be acceptable for healthcare personnel. To alleviate this issue for future crises, the FDA could consider a separate 510(k) requirement that allows manufacturers to market any appropriate NIOSH-certified respirator during an influenza pandemic. This would rapidly allow all certified respirators to be available for use by healthcare personnel.

LESSONS LEARNED FROM 2009 H1N1 POLICIES RELEVANT TO PPE FOR HEALTHCARE PERSONNEL

The arrival of novel H1N1 influenza A in 2009 was accompanied by a number of policy questions relevant to PPE. The lack of precise information about the modes of influenza transmission, the contagiousness, the virulence of novel H1N1 influenza A, the at-risk population, and the efficacy of different devices in preventing transmission led to a variety of recommendations at different times by federal and local government public health agencies. Delayed and/or disparate recommendations often led to confusion among healthcare personnel and their employers, who had to decide what to tell personnel about what type of PPE to wear and when. In addition, little research was available to guide health system officials in making decisions about the quantities of various types of PPE needed to protect their workforce. A major problem encountered was a slow response in tailoring recommendations as more knowledge about virulence and affected populations became available.

The committee looked to two examples of response to 2009 H1N1 (New York City [NYC] and Northern Virginia), with information provided by committee members, workshop speakers, and individual interviews. Northern Virginia hospitals, for example, developed standardized infection control policies that included a definition of high-risk workers. To address supply chain shortfalls, the 14 member hospitals of the Northern Virginia Hospital Alliance (NVHA) agreed to follow CDC respirator guidelines until no longer practical. As a matter of practice, hospitals modified the CDC guidelines in regards to PPE requirements for non-high-risk workers, especially as it became clear in fall 2009 that the virulence of 2009 H1N1 was similar to seasonal influenza viruses (Personal communication, Zachary Corrigan, NVHA, 2010).

In NYC, the fire department emphasized the need for paramedics and emergency medical technicians to use N95 respirators as they work in the pre-hospital environment where environmental controls do not exist. When the H1N1 virus first emerged, the NYC Department of Health and Mental Hygiene and the New York State department of health initially recommended N95 respirators but then scaled back the recommendations to face masks to be consistent with seasonal influenza recommendations once it was determined that the virulence and transmissibility were similar to seasonal influenza. However, once CDC published its interim infection control guidance in October 2009, the New York city and state departments of health revised their guidance to be consistent with the federal recommendations for N95 respirators. In anticipation of the second wave of H1N1 returning in Fall 2009, the city health department, working with the NYC Office of Emergency Management, convened regular healthcare emergency planning meetings to improve hospital and primary care preparedness. The NYC health department also put in place a program to provide additional N95 respirators from a local government stockpile for healthcare facilities experiencing supply shortages during the 2009 pandemic (Personal communication, David Prezant, New York City Fire Department).

PPE Policies During the Novel H1N1 Influenza Pandemic

During the initial phase of the 2009 H1N1 influenza pandemic, infection control guidelines from some of the major public health organizations differed, primarily as related to respiratory protection (Table 5-1). The World Health Organization (WHO) recommended standard and droplet precautions (including a face mask, a gown, gloves, eye protection, and hand hygiene) for those working in direct contact with patients, and additional precautions for aerosol-generating procedures, including wearing a facial particulate respirator (WHO, 2009). The WHO recommendations took into account the need for sustainability in a variety of countries and encouraged each country to issue its own guidelines. CDC recommended a fit tested, disposable N95 respirator or better for healthcare personnel who enter the rooms of patients in isolation with suspected or confirmed novel H1N1 influenza (CDC, 2009b). For emergency medical responders, CDC recommended a fit tested, disposable N95 respirator for those personnel "who are in close contact" with patients with confirmed or suspected 2009 H1N1, for personnel "engaged in aerosol generating activities," and for personnel involved in the "interfacility transfer" of patients with suspected or confirmed 2009 H1N1 (CDC, 2009a). The Public Health Agency of Canada used a tiered approach that recommended N95 use for aerosol-generating procedures with direct patient contact only (PHAC, 2009a,b,c,d).

Overview of Recent Policy Research

Research on healthcare policies and their implementation is lacking as it pertains to the use of PPE. Given the many PPE policy issues during

TABLE 5-1 Overview of 2009–2010 H1N1 Policies and Practices Regarding Personal Protective Equipment and H1N1 Influenza

	CDC Guidance 4/29/09 Novel Pandemic Influenza	CDC Guidance 10/15/09 Novel Pandemic Influenza	CDC Guidance for Seasonal Influenza 9/20/10	WHO Guidance	Public Health Agency of Canada Guidance for Novel H1N1
Recommended level of infection control precautions	Standard and contact precautions and eye protection	Standard and droplet precautions	Adhere to standard and droplet precautions	Standard and droplet precautions	Tiered approach
Recommended respiratory PPE	NIOSH-certified N95 respirator	NIOSH-certified N95 respirator	Face mask except for aerosol-generating procedures, use N95 or better	Face mask except for aerosol-generating procedures	Face mask except for aerosol-generating procedures
Did the respiratory PPE recommendation differ by work task?	Yes—direct care versus indirect patient contact	Yes—direct care versus indirect patient contact	Yes—direct care versus aerosol-generating procedures	Yes	Yes

NOTE: CDC = Centers for Disease Control and Prevention; NIOSH = National Institute for Occupational Safety and Health; PPE = personal protective equipment; WHO = World Health Organization.
SOURCES: CDC (2009a,b); PHAC (2009a,b,c,d); WHO (2009).

the initial stages of 2009 H1N1, more papers are likely to be forthcoming as healthcare institutions document their experiences and researchers have the opportunity to publish their findings. This section reviews some of the research and summaries published since 2007 regarding policies on PPE use. Because PPE is one part of infection control strategies, some of the communications and emergency planning aspects are part of a larger discussion on pandemic planning (see, e.g., Daugherty et al., 2010).

Supplies of PPE

One issue faced during 2009 H1N1 was ensuring that healthcare facilities had adequate supplies of PPE and other supplies. As noted in an article by Rebmann and Wagner (2009), less than a month after the first case of laboratory-confirmed novel H1N1 was reported in the United States, CDC had deployed 25 percent of the Strategic National Stockpile (SNS) of N95 respirators. A focus group study of infection control specialists identified issues faced in the first months of the pandemic (Rebmann and Wagner, 2009). Supply issues of prime concern included running out of respirators or certain sizes of respirators and facing back orders early in the pandemic. Similar supply issues were seen in the early months of the pandemic in Australia, with concerns noted about the amount of time and quantity of PPE supplies retrieved from the SNS (Eizenberg, 2009).

Determining the quantities of PPE required was the focus of a report by Murray and colleagues (2010) that examined the use of facial protective equipment from late June through mid-December 2009 in three Vancouver, Canada, hospitals. During that time, 865 patients with suspected cases of H1N1 influenza were admitted, with 149 patients having laboratory-confirmed H1N1 influenza infection; 134,281 masks and 173,145 N95 respirators were used. Comparisons were made of the number of respirators, masks, and protective eyewear used within the same period in 2008, with increases of 107 percent in the number of respirators, 70 percent in the number of eyewear, and 196 percent in the number of masks. The authors reported that the Ministry of Health plans for pandemic influenza called for hospitals to have a 10-week supply of PPE equipment, but they did not account for increases in the supplies that would be needed.

Two reports provide detailed descriptions of the planning process used by the U.S. Department of Veterans Affairs to determine the quantities and types of PPE needed to respond to pandemic influenza. This process included considerations of many factors that weighed into those decisions, such as the anticipated number of patients, the number of healthcare worker contacts per patient, PPE needs, and cost (Koenig et al., 2007; Radonovich et al., 2009).

The Northern Virginia Regional Hospital Coordinating Center, the operational arm of the Northern Virginia Hospital Allliance Emergency Preparedness and Response Program, reported that member hospitals developed regional stockpiles of respiratory PPE based on a risk stratification of their personnel. They used OSHA's occupational risk pyramid for pandemic influenza to estimate the numbers of personnel at higher risk and then used a formula that considered the size of the facility and the number of providers to get final estimates for distribution. Supplies of PAPRs, reusable elastomeric N95 respirators, disposable N95 respirators, and surgical masks were provided to member hospitals from regional stockpiles (Personal communication, Zachary Corrigan, NVHA, 2010).

Several studies have made initial attempts to estimate the quantity of PPE needed, but further work on predictive models is needed. Swaminathan and colleagues (2007) conducted a simulation study in nine Australian hospital emergency departments designed to evaluate the number of contacts between patients and healthcare personnel and to determine the number of types of PPE that would be required. Compliance of healthcare personnel in using the appropriate PPE was also examined. The study focused on only the first 6 hours of contact[1] with a suspected case. The researchers reported an average of 12 close contacts, with 19 exposures per "case," and estimated that approximately 20 N95 respirators, 22 gowns, and 25 gloves would have been required to protect healthcare personnel during the first 6 hours of care. Given the rates of compliance noted in this study, up to 40 percent of healthcare personnel may have required post-exposure prophylaxis. This study provides some initial objective evidence regarding the numbers of PPE sets that might be required, but it was limited by its short duration of only 6 hours and by the simulation of a patient who was not critically ill. Similar types of research that extend the observation duration and simulate more severe illness would be helpful in estimating PPE requirements.

In Japan, Hashikura and Kizu (2009) used the severe acute respiratory syndrome outbreak as a paradigm for PPE use. The researchers re-

---

[1]Close contact was defined as being within 1 meter of a patient or within an isolation room.

viewed the literature and the guidelines on PPE use from many countries, and then estimated the numbers of PPE ensembles that would be required during a pandemic, using information on the type of pandemic, type of healthcare worker, and numbers of PPE ensembles per classification per day. They estimated (using OSHA recommendations) that four sets (N95, gloves, gowns, and goggles) would be used per day by high-risk healthcare personnel, who are defined as persons performing high-risk procedures, such as intubations, suctioning, and manipulating respiratory equipment. Two sets of appropriate PPE was the estimate for medium- and low-risk healthcare personnel (this included an N95 respirator for medium-risk and a surgical mask for low-risk workers). The researchers also estimated that two surgical masks would be required for every in-patient and one for every out-patient. They then estimated the total numbers of PPE required for a 300-bed hospital during an 8-week pandemic— nearly 20,000 N95 respirators, 122,000 surgical masks, 21,000 goggles and gowns, and 172,000 pairs of gloves would be needed. This study provides an initial start on the question of estimated quantities, but is theoretical and based only on published recommendation guidelines. The methodology is logical, but needs to be validated. Data on actual use of PPE by a hospital is needed to compare the accuracy of the predictions.

A study comparing single-use versus reusable surgical gowns high-lights another area of discussion regarding costs and quantity of supplies. Baykasoglu and colleagues (2009) conducted a cost/benefit study that considered a number of factors, including laundry, sterilization, and waste disposal costs, as well as the extent of protection and functionality. The study determined that the single-use sets had higher benefits, but when costs were considered, the more expensive reusable sets had higher benefit/cost ratios. This area of research and modeling could provide practical insights, particularly as effective decontamination processes become defined.

H1N1 Experiences with Use of PPE by Healthcare Personnel

Evidence of transmission to healthcare personnel was reported during the pandemic, indicating the need for comprehensive PPE policies. Santos and colleagues (2010) examined an NYC hospital's absentee records for 3 months (April through June 2009) and compared the results with the same periods in 2007 and 2008. The researchers found that healthcare personnel in the adult and pediatric emergency departments had the highest infection rate per department. The peak of influenza in healthcare personnel was noted to have lagged slightly behind the peak in the general public.

The literature on policies put in place during 2009 H1N1 will likely grow in the next several years. At this point only a few articles have been published that focus on PPE use during the initial phases of H1N1. Early in the epidemic, Perez-Padilla and colleagues (2009) reported their experience in Mexico City. They focused on the clinical presentation of H1N1, but also noted information on the transmission of disease to healthcare personnel. The report noted that 22 of 190 workers who became infected had been involved in caring for the first 3 H1N1 patients in a series of 18 patients admitted during the first month of the pandemic in spring 2009. These included 19 out of 104 emergency department workers who had been within 2 meters of a patient or had direct contact with a patient. These 22 workers had mild to moderate disease, and none required hospitalization. The hospital then instituted strict infection control measures, including N95s, gowns, gloves, goggles, and hand hygiene, and noted that no additional workers became ill with influenza-like illness, although 26 did have varied respiratory symptoms and were treated with oseltamavir.

Focus group discussions with a group of infection preventionists in the United States pointed out the logistical issues that were faced in the first months of the pandemic in trying to fit test a large number of staff (Rebmann and Wagner, 2009) as well as the challenges in determining whether and when to recommend the use of face masks or respirators. Of the focus group participants, approximately one-third said that PPE-use guidelines changed at their facilities about halfway through the event.

A survey of healthcare epidemiologists, administrators, and other members of the Society for Healthcare Epidemiology of America in May 2009 found that 19.3 percent of respondents strongly agreed and 52.7 percent agreed that "the recommendation for airborne precautions for suspected H1N1 cases was appropriate at the beginning of the H1N1 crisis" at his or her institution (Lautenbach et al., 2010, p. 3). When asked whether airborne precautions for suspected cases were appropriate throughout the H1N1 crisis, 7.5 percent strongly agreed and 17.5 percent agreed. Supplies of N95s were a concern with some respondents; 16.9 percent disagreed and 8.8 percent strongly disagreed with the statement that "N95 masks were readily available throughout the H1N1 crisis at my institution" (Lautenbach et al., 2010, p. 3).

Changes in PPE guidelines were an issue for healthcare personnel in Australia, as identified in a questionnaire and focus group study (Corley et al., 2010). Healthcare staff reported confusion over the changing requirements and noted that this led to staff feeling "undervalued" and "unprotected." Discomfort in wearing a respirator for a 12-hour shift with maybe a 1- to 1.5-hour break was noted as a challenge, as was the considerable amount of time spent on donning and doffing PPE.

The need to reinforce education and communication about PPE and other infection control processes for pre-hospital healthcare personnel, including paramedics, was noted as one of the key lessons learned in the H1N1 pandemic by a group reviewing the response in Victoria, Australia (Smith et al., 2009).

Prior to the 2009 H1N1 pandemic, simulations and other planning efforts included a focus on PPE issues and policies. Phin and colleagues (2009) assessed a 24-hour simulation exercise in England and highlighted PPE cost and procurement issues as well as issues involving the storage of PPE supplies and increases in the amount of trash generated. The exercise noted unnecessary staff movement related to delivery of supplies and provision of services that also impacted PPE use. A review of emergency plans in three Ontario hospitals noted a number of PPE issues, including addressing fit testing requirements; regular training, including practice drills; stockpiling, warehousing, and inventory management; and storage and maintenance of PPE (Amaratunga et al., 2007). An extensive planning effort by a task force of the European Society of Intensive Care Medicine addressed a range of policy issues related to pandemic planning, including the need to develop protocols for safe performance of procedures (including aerosol-generating procedures) that might put personnel at risk (Sprung et al., 2010). Training regarding PPE and an organizational culture that promotes safety were also discussed.

SUMMARY OF PROGRESS

Preparations and implementation of infection control plans for 2009 H1N1 influenza brought into sharp focus the efforts by healthcare professionals, emergency planners, professional associations, healthcare facilities, policy makers, government agencies, labor unions, and others to address PPE policies and logistics. Articles continue to be published on the recent experience and the challenges and successes in providing face masks, respirators, and other PPE to healthcare personnel. As lessons learned during that experience continue to add to the body of knowledge, incorporating this information into research, policy, and practice efforts will be important. In the initial phases of an epidemic or pandemic—when there are many unknowns about the virus or agent—one of the challenges is to determine PPE policy and then to adapt those policies as information is gained on the severity, transmission, and nature of the disease with an emphasis on communicating those changes. Standards-setting, regulatory, training, and research efforts continue to move toward improved respiratory protection, and recent work has begun to focus on the specifics of how to tailor PPE devices and PPE training to address the specific needs of healthcare personnel.

FINDINGS AND RESEARCH NEEDS

This chapter has provided an overview of the many policy and regulatory issues relevant to developing and improving PPE for healthcare personnel. The committee's findings (outlined in Box 5-2) and research needs and recommendations (below) point to the many opportunities available, making now a particularly urgent time to build on recent experiences and needs and to move forward with the policy research and regulatory changes that will improve protection for healthcare personnel.

The committee highlights the following research needs:

- **Lessons learned from the 2009 H1N1 policies relevant to PPE:** Case studies of the implementation of 2009 H1N1 PPE-related policies should be gathered and evaluated.
- **PPE supply estimates:** Studies are needed that compare theoretical models of estimating quantities of PPE for emergency preparedness with recent experience to inform future public health planning.
- **Cost-effectiveness research:** Research is needed into cost-effectiveness issues relevant to PPE, including issues of disposable and reusable equipment.
- **Impact of public health guidance:** Prospective research efforts should examine the impact of public health guidance on PPE compliance by state, local, and health system policy; clinical practice; and costs.

BOX 5-2
Findings

- Public health guidance regarding personal protective equipment (PPE) use for protection from novel viral respiratory infections needs to be timely, flexible, and consistent and should require the appropriate PPE based on what is known at the time about transmission and virulence.
- Public health policy regarding PPE use for healthcare personnel's protection from viral respiratory infections needs to recognize that transmission occurs in the community from family and friends as well as in the work environment from patients and coworkers. Recognition of this fact is the foundation for an aggressive vaccination program for healthcare personnel.

RECOMMENDATIONS

Recommendation: Move Forward on Better Fitting Respirators
NPPTL should continue rulemaking processes for TIL regulations that require respirators to meet fit criteria. To improve consumer and purchaser information on fit capabilities, NIOSH should establish a website to disseminate fit test results for specific respirator models on an anthropometric (NIOSH) test panel, where such data exist.

Recommendation: Clarify PPE Guidelines for Outbreaks of Novel Viral Respiratory Infections
NIOSH, other CDC divisions, OSHA, and other public health agencies should develop a coordinated process to make, announce, and revise consistent guidelines regarding the use of PPE to be worn by healthcare personnel during a verified, sustained national/international outbreak of a novel viral respiratory infection. The agencies should tailor their guidance in a timely and coordinated manner as the virulence, contagiousness, and affected populations are further characterized.

Recommendation: Standards and Certification for Face Masks and Face Shields
NIOSH, OSHA, and standards-development organizations should develop the standards and certification processes

needed to assess the performance of face masks and face shields as PPE. The development of standards and certification processes should be guided by research regarding their efficacy as PPE.

- OSHA and CDC should clarify that face masks are governed by the general PPE standard (29 CFR 1910.132) and not by the respiratory protection standard (29 CFR 1910.134).
- NIOSH should work with other agencies and standards-setting organizations to develop voluntary consensus standards and independent third-party testing and certification processes for face shields and face masks, with specific tests for assessing prevention of transmission of viral respiratory diseases.

Recommendation: Establish PPE Regulations for Healthcare Personnel
CDC, including NIOSH, and OSHA should develop and promulgate guidelines and regulations that are consistent regarding the use of PPE by healthcare personnel for influenza and other viral respiratory diseases:

- To assist employers in complying with the OSHA PPE standard, OSHA should specify the voluntary consensus standards that are required to be met for non-respirator PPE (e.g., gowns, gloves, face shields, face masks) in the event of influenza and other viral respiratory diseases.
- OSHA, with input from CDC and other agencies and organizations, should work toward promulgating an aerosol-transmissible diseases standard that would include prevention of the transmission of influenza and other viral respiratory diseases.

As noted throughout the chapters, this report is an update of a prior IOM report. In surveying the landscape of research that has been conducted since the 2008 report and even in the wake of the 2009 H1N1 influenza pandemic, the committee was struck by the lack of urgency in addressing the basic, applied, and clinical research questions that, if answered, would go a long way toward improving preparedness and prevention against future influenza epidemics and pandemics and outbreaks of other respiratory viral agents. Looking back is often a way to propel efforts in moving forward. The committee hopes that this review will jumpstart and strengthen improvements in PPE for healthcare personnel that could be relevant to a range of viral respiratory diseases.

REFERENCES

Amaratunga, C. A., T. L. O'Sullivan, K. P. Phillips, L. Lemyre, E. O'Connor, D. Dow, and W. Corneil. 2007. Ready, aye ready? Support mechanisms for healthcare workers in emergency planning: A critical gap analysis of three hospital emergency plans. *American Journal of Disaster Medicine* 2(4):195-210.

ASTM International. 2010a. *ASTM WK27438: New specification for antimicrobial medical gloves.* http://www.astm.org/WorkItems/WK27438.htm (accessed November 11, 2010).

———. 2010b. *Product certification.* http://www.astm.org/SNEWS/MJ_2010/f2350_mj10.html (accessed December 8, 2010).

———. 2010c. *Standardization news: Antimicrobial medical gloves.* http://www.astm.org/SNEWS/MJ_2010/d1140_mj10.html (accessed November 29, 2010).

Baykasoglu, A., T. Dereli, and N. Yilankirkan. 2009. Application of cost/benefit analysis for surgical gown and drape selection: A case study. *American Journal of Infection Control* 37(3):215-226.

California Code of Regulations. 2010. *Title 8, Section 5199: Aerosol transmissible diseases standard.* http://www.dir.ca.gov/title8/5199.html (accessed November 11, 2010).

CDC (Centers for Disease Control and Prevention). 2009a. *Interim guidance for emergency medical services (EMS) systems and 9-1-1 public safety answering points (PSAPs) for management of patients with confirmed or suspected swine-origin influenza A (H1N1) infection.* http://cdc.gov/h1n1flu/guidance_ems.htm (accessed December 8, 2010).

———. 2009b. *Interim guidance on infection control measures for 2009 H1N1 influenza in healthcare settings, including protection of healthcare personnel.* http://cdc.gov/h1n1flu/guidelines_infection_control.htm (accessed December 8, 2010).

———. 2010. *Prevention strategies for seasonal influenza in healthcare settings.* http://www.cdc.gov/flu/professionals/infectioncontrol/healthcaresettings.htm (accessed December 8, 2010).

Corley, A., N. E. Hammond, and J. F. Fraser. 2010. The experiences of health care workers employed in an Australian intensive care unit during the H1N1 influenza pandemic of 2009: A phenomenological study. *International Journal of Nursing Studies* 47(5):577-585.

Daugherty, E. L., A. L. Carlson, and T. M. Perl. 2010. Healthcare epidemiology: Planning for the inevitable: Preparing for epidemic and pandemic respiratory illness in the shadow of H1N1 influenza. *Clinical Infectious Diseases* 50(8):1145-1154.

Eizenberg, P. 2009. The general practice experience of the swine flu epidemic in Victoria—lessons from the front line. *Medical Journal of Australia* 191(3):151-153.

Hashikura, M., and J. Kizu. 2009. Stockpile of personal protective equipment in hospital settings: Preparedness for influenza pandemics. *American Journal of Infection Control* 37(9):703-707.

IOM (Institute of Medicine). 2008. *Preparing for an influenza pandemic: Personal protective equipment for healthcare workers.* Washington, DC: The National Academies Press.

———. 2010. *Certifying personal protective technologies: Improving worker safety.* Washington, DC: The National Academies Press.

Jensen, P. A., L. A. Lambert, M. F. Iademarco, and R. Ridzon. 2005. Guidelines for preventing the transmission of mycobacterium tuberculosis in health-care settings, 2005. *MMWR Recommendations and Reports* 54(RR-17):1-141.

Koenig, K. L., C. J. Boatright, J. A. Hancock, F. J. Denny, D. S. Teeter, C. A. Kahn, and C. H. Schultz. 2007. Health care facilities' "war on terrorism": A deliberate process for recommending personal protective equipment. *American Journal of Emergency Medicine* 25(2):185-195.

Lautenbach, E., S. Saint, D. K. Henderson, and A. D. Harris. 2010. Initial response of health care institutions to emergence of H1N1 influenza: Experiences, obstacles, and perceived future needs. *Clinical Infectious Diseases* 50(4):523-527.

Murray, M., J. Grant, E. Bryce, P. Chilton, and L. Forrester. 2010. Facial protective equipment, personnel, and pandemics: Impact of the pandemic (H1N1) 2009 virus on personnel and use of facial protective equipment. *Infection Control and Hospital Epidemiology* 31(10):1011-1016.

NIOSH (National Institute for Occupational Safety and Health). 2010a. *NIOSH docket 137: Total inward leakage requirements for half-mask air-purifying particulate respirators.* http://www.cdc.gov/niosh/docket/archive/docket137.html (accessed November 11, 2010).

———. 2010b. *NIOSH investigation of 3M model 8000 filtering facepiece respirators as requested by the California Occupational Safety and Health Administration, Division of Occupational Safety and Health. HETA 2010-0044-3109.* http://cdc.gov/niosh/hhe/reports/pdfs/2010-0044-3109.pdf (accessed December 8, 2010).

OSHA (Occupational Safety and Health Administration). 2007. Employer payment for personal protective equipment; final rule. *Federal Register* 72(220):64341-64430.

————. 2009. Updating OSHA standards based on national consensus standards; personal protective equipment. *Federal Register* 74(173):46350-64430.

————. 2010. Infectious diseases. *Federal Register* 75(87):24835-24844.

Perez-Padilla, R., D. de la Rosa-Zamboni, S. P. de Leon, M. Hernandez, F. Quinones-Falconi, E. Bautista, A. Ramirez-Venegas, J. Rojas-Serrano, C. E. Ormsby, A. Corrales, A. Higuera, E. Mondragon, J. A. Cordova-Villalobos, and the INER Working Group on Influenza. 2009. Pneumonia and respiratory failure from swine-origin influenza A (H1N1) in Mexico. *New England Journal of Medicine* 361(7):680-689.

PHAC (Public Health Agency of Canada). 2009a. *Guidance: Infection prevention and control measures for health care workers in acute care facilities.* http://www.phac-aspc.gc.ca/alert-alerte/h1n1/hp-ps/ig_acf-ld_esa-eng.php (accessed December 8, 2010).

————. 2009b. *Guidance: Infection prevention and control measures for health care workers in long-term care facilities.* http://www.phac-aspc.gc.ca/alert-alerte/h1n1/hp-ps/prevention-eng.php (accessed December 8, 2010).

————. 2009c. *Guidance: Infection prevention and control measures for pre-hospital care.* http://www.phac-aspc.gc.ca/alert-alerte/h1n1/hp-ps/pc-sp-eng.php (accessed December 8, 2010).

————. 2009d. *Point of care risk assessment tool for pandemic (H1N1) 2009 flu virus.* http://www.hsabc.org/webuploads/files/h1n1/CNV_1_765_Point_of_Care_Risk_Assessment_Tool_for_Pandemic.pdf (accessed December 8, 2010).

Phin, N. F., A. J. Rylands, J. Allan, C. Edwards, J. E. Enstone, and J. S. Nguyen-Van-Tam. 2009. Personal protective equipment in an influenza pandemic: A UK simulation exercise. *Journal of Hospital Infection* 71(1):15-21.

Radonovich, L. J., P. D. Magalian, M. K. Hollingsworth, and G. Baracco. 2009. Stockpiling supplies for the next influenza pandemic. *Emerging Infectious Diseases* 5(6):June.

Rebmann, T., and W. Wagner. 2009. Infection preventionists' experience during the first months of the 2009 novel H1N1 influenza A pandemic. *American Journal of Infection Control* 37(10):e5-e16.

Santos, C. D., R. B. Bristow, and J. V. Vorenkamp. 2010. Which health care workers were most affected during the spring 2009 H1N1 pandemic? *Disaster Medicine and Public Health Preparedness* 4(1):47-54.

Siegel, J., E. Rhinehart, M. Jackson, L. Chiarello, and the Healthcare Infection Control Practices Advisory Committee. 2007. *2007 guideline for isolation precautions: Preventing transmission of infectious agents in healthcare settings.* http://www.cdc.gov/hicpac/pdf/isolation/Isolation2007.pdf (accessed November 16, 2010).

Smith, E. C., F. M. Burkle, Jr., P. F. Holman, J. M. Dunlop, and F. L. Archer. 2009. Lessons from the front lines: The prehospital experience of the 2009 novel H1N1 outbreak in Victoria, Australia. *Disaster Medicine and Public Health Preparedness* 3(Suppl. 2):S154-S159.

Sprung, C., J. Zimmerman, M. Christian, G. Joynt, J. Hick, B. Taylor, G. Richards, C. Sandrock, R. Cohen, and B. Adini. 2010. Recommendations for intensive care unit and hospital preparations for an influenza epidemic or mass disaster: Summary report of the European Society of Intensive Care Medicine's task force for intensive care unit triage during an influenza epidemic or mass disaster. *Intensive Care Medicine* 36(3):428-443.

Swaminathan, A., R. Martin, S. Gamon, C. Aboltins, E. Athan, G. Braitberg, M. G. Catton, L. Cooley, D. E. Dwyer, D. Edmonds, D. P. Eisen, K. Hosking, A. J. Hughes, P. D. Johnson, A. V. Maclean, M. O'Reilly, S. E. Peters, R. L. Stuart, R. Moran, and M. L. Grayson. 2007. Personal protective equipment and antiviral drug use during hospitalization for suspected avian or pandemic influenza. *Emerging Infectious Diseases* 13(10):1541-1547.

WHO (World Health Organization). 2009. *Infection prevention and control in health care for confirmed or suspected cases of pandemic (H1N1) 2009 and influenza-like illnesses.* http://www.who.int/csr/resources/publications/ SwineInfluenza_infectioncontrol.pdf (accessed December 8, 2010).

A

Workshop Agenda

The National Academy of Sciences
Board Room
2100 C Street, NW
Washington, DC

Meeting Agenda

Thursday, February 25, 2010

11:00 a.m. **Welcome and Introductions**
Elaine Larson, Committee Chair

Sponsor's Charge to the Committee and Background Information
Maryann D'Alessandro, Associate Director for Science, National Personal Protective Technology Laboratory (NPPTL), National Institute for Occupational Safety and Health (NIOSH)
Les Boord, Director, NPPTL, NIOSH
David Weissman, NIOSH Healthcare Program Manager
Roland Berry Ann, Deputy Director, NPPTL

Discussion

12:45 p.m. **Lunch**

1:30 p.m. **Context for the Study**

1:30–2:30   Current NPPTL Research on Personal Protective
            Equipment (PPE) and Influenza
            Ron Shaffer, NPPTL

            Discussion

2:30–3:30   Project B.R.E.A.T.H.E. and the Respiratory
            Protection Clinical Effectiveness Trial
            Lewis Radonovich, Director, National Center for
            Occupational Health and Infection Control,
            Veterans Health Administration

            Discussion

3:30 p.m.   Adjourn

Institute of Medicine
Current Research Issues—Personal Protective Equipment for
Healthcare Workers to Prevent Transmission of Pandemic Influenza
and Other Viral Respiratory Infections

WORKSHOP

Venable Conference Center
575 Seventh Street, NW
Capitol Room–Eighth Floor
Washington, DC

Thursday, June 3, 2010

Objectives:
- Provide an overview of recent research (2007–2010)
- Identify lessons learned from the 2009–2010 H1N1 pandemic relevant to PPE for healthcare workers
- Identify research gaps and directions needed for future research

8:00 a.m.   Welcome and Opening Remarks
            Elaine Larson, Chair, Committee on Personal Protective
            Equipment for Healthcare Workers to Prevent
            Transmission of Pandemic Influenza and Other Viral
            Respiratory Infections: Current Research Issues

8:15 a.m.   **Panel 1: Research on Influenza Transmission**
Facilitators: Peter Palese, Allison Aiello

        8:15–8:30   Update on animal studies
                         Daniel Perez, University of Maryland
        8:30–8:45   Update on environmental monitoring studies
                         Bill Lindsley, NIOSH
        8:45–9:00   Update on aerosol-dispersion modeling studies
                         Mark Nicas, University of California–Berkeley
        9:00–9:15   Update on nosocomial transmission studies
                         Caroline Breese Hall, University of Rochester
        9:15–9:30   Update on human challenge studies
                         Jonathan Van-Tam, University of Nottingham
        9:30–10:00 Discussion with the committee

10:00 a.m.   **Panel 2: Research on Advances in PPE Technology**
Facilitators: Karen Coyne, Howard Cohen, Ken Gall, Bill
Kojola

        10:00–10:25 Update on mask and respirator technology
                         Lisa Brosseau, University of Minnesota
        10:25–10:40 Update on PPE performance in preventing
                         influenza transmission
                         Joe Wander, U.S. Air Force
        10:40–10:55 Update on human interface research and
                         materials technology
                         Sundaresan Jayaraman, Georgia Institute of
                         Technology
        10:55–11:10 Update on face shield/eye protection technology
                         Gilad Shoham, Medonyx, Inc.
        11:10–11:25 Update on gown and glove technology
                         Vicki Barbur, Cardinal Health
        11:25–12:00 Discussion with the committee

12:00 p.m.   **Lunch**

12:45 p.m.   **Panel 3: PPE Implementation—Observational and
Clinical Studies**
Facilitators: Richard Wenzel, Allison McGeer, and Bob Cohen

        12:45–1:00   Observational studies on PPE use by healthcare
                         workers and barriers to use
                         Annalee Yassi, University of British Columbia

1:00–1:15	Implementation of PPE programs in California during the 2009–2010 flu season Robert Harrison, University of California–San Francisco
1:15–1:30	Update on clinical studies Trish Perl, Johns Hopkins University
1:30–1:45	Proposed clinical study Lewis Radonovich, U.S. Department of Veterans Affairs
1:45–2:15	Discussion with the committee

2:15 p.m.   **Panel 4: PPE Implementation—Individual and Organizational Studies**
Facilitators: Bonnie Rogers and David DeJoy

2:15–2:30	Update on research on organizations and worker safety culture David Hofmann, University of North Carolina
2:30–2:45	Update on research on organizational and team learning Ingrid Nembhard, Yale University
2:45–3:00	Dental community experience John Molinari, University of Detroit
3:00–3:15	Update on research on home and community healthcare workers' use of PPE Ruth Ann Ellison, Apria Healthcare
3:15–3:45	Discussion with the committee

3:45 p.m.   **Panel 5: PPE Implementation—International and U.S. Policy Research Perspective on the H1N1 Experience with PPE**
Facilitators: Gloria Addo-Ayensu and David Prezant

3:45–4:00	Australia's experience with H1N1 and PPE Dominic Dwyer, Westmead Hospital (via phone)
4:00–4:15	Mexico's experience with H1N1 and PPE Rogelio Perez-Padilla, Instituto Nacional de Enfermedades Respiratorias (via phone)
4:15–4:30	New York City's experience with H1N1 and PPE Marcelle Layton, New York City Department of Health and Mental Hygiene
4:30–4:45	Update on policy research David Henderson, National Institutes of Health
4:45–5:15	Discussion with the committee

5:15 p.m.   **Public Comment—Registered Speakers** (3 minutes per speaker)
Moderator, Elaine Larson

- Gamunu Wijetunge, National Highway Traffic Safety Administration
- Donald Milton, University of Maryland
- Nicole McCullough, 3M
- Kathy Robinson, National Association of State EMS Officials
- Eileen Storey, NIOSH
- Robert Guidos, Infectious Diseases Society of America
- William Borwegen, Service Employees International Union
- Judene Bartley, Epidemiology Consulting Services, APIC Representative
- Padma Natarajan, Infectious Diseases Society of America
- Leslie McGorman, Infectious Diseases Society of America
- Korlu Kuyon, Maryland Department of Health and Mental Hygiene, Perkins Hospital Center

6:00 p.m.   **Summary**
Howard Cohen and Richard Wenzel

6:15 p.m.   **Adjourn**

B

Participants List

Gloria Addo-Ayensu
Director
Fairfax County Department of
Health

Allison E. Aiello
John G. Searle Assistant Professor
of Public Health
University of Michigan School of
Public Health

Darryl Alexander
Program Director
American Federation of Teachers,
AFL–CIO

Jennylynn Balmer
Employee Safety Programs
Administrator
Inova Health System

Evelyn Balogun
Medical Director
Temple University Hospital

Vicki Barbur
Vice President, R&D
Clinician Apparel and Patient
Protection
Cardinal Health

Judene Bartley
Vice President, Epidemiology
Consulting Services, Inc.
APIC Representative

Jo Anne Bennett
New York City Department of
Health and Mental Hygiene

Joseph Beres
Industrial Hygienist
U.S. Department of State

Kim Biedermann
GlaxoSmithKline

Werner Bischoff
Assistant Professor, Internal
Medicine
Assistant Hospital Epidemiologist
Wake Forest University Health
Sciences

William Borwegen
Occupational Health and Safety
Director
Service Employees International
Union

Katie Brewer
Senior Policy Analyst
American Nurses Association

Lisa M. Brosseau
Associate Professor
University of Minnesota School of
  Public Health

Gavin Burdge
Industrial Hygienist
BMT Designers and Planners, Inc.

Karen Caine
Department of Health and Human
  Services

Leigh Chapman
Infection Prevention Coordinator
St. Joseph Medical Center

Elizabeth F. Claverie-Williams
Senior Microbiology Reviewer
Senior Regulatory Reviewer
Food and Drug Administration

Howard J. Cohen
Professor Emeritus
University of New Haven

Robert Cohen
Director, Pulmonary and Critical
  Care Medicine, Cook County
  Health and Hospitals System
Stroger Hospital of Cook County

Matt Conlon
Vice President, Market
  Development
Cantel Medical Corp

Katherine Cox
Director, Health and Safety
  Program
American Federation of State,
  County, and Municipal
  Employees International

Karen Coyne
Research General Engineer
U.S. Army Edgewood Chemical
  Biologic Center

Mae Cundiff
Infection Control Preventionist
Providence Hospital

Terrell Cunningham
Scientific Reviewer
Food and Drug Administration

Maryann D'Alessandro
Associate Director for Science
National Personal Protective
  Technology Laboratory
National Institute for Occupational
  Safety and Health

John Decker
Senior Scientist
National Institute for Occupational
  Safety and Health

Enjoli DeGrasse
Industrial Hygienist
International Brotherhood of
  Teamsters

David M. DeJoy
Professor
Department of Health Promotion
  and Behavior
College of Public Health
University of Georgia

Steve Duff
Sales Manager
LM Gerson

Dominic E. Dwyer
Medical Virologist
Centre for Infectious Diseases and
    Microbiology
Institute of Clinical Pathology and
    Medical Research
Westmead Hospital, Australia

Ruth Ann Ellison
Vice President
Clinical Regulatory Compliance
Apria Healthcare, Inc.

Judy Estep
Program Associate
Institute of Medicine

June Fisher
Physician/Director
Training for Development of
    Innovative Control Technologies
    Project

Ken Gall
Professor
School of Materials Science and
    Engineering
Petit Institute of Bioengineering
    and Bioscience
Georgia Institute of Technology

Jackie Galluzzo
Infection Prevention and Control
    Practitioner
St. Joseph Medical Center

Bruce Gellin
Director, National Vaccine
    Program Office
Department of Health and Human
    Services

George Gentile
Medical and First Responder
    Program Manager
Department of Homeland Security

TroyJennene Gibbs
Health and Safety Officer
City of Alexandria, VA, Fire
    Department

Marta Gill
Montgomery County
Department of Health and Human
    Services
Public Health Emergency
    Preparedness and Response
    Program

Joelle Glass
Infection Preventionist
Sinai Hospital

Daniel Glucksman
Public Affairs Director
International Safety Equipment
    Association

Robert Guidos
Vice President, Public Policy and
    Government Relations
Infectious Diseases Society of
    America

Caroline Breese Hall
Professor of Pediatrics and
    Medicine
University of Rochester School of
    Medicine

Elise Handelman
Occupational Safety and Health
   Administration

Sarah Hanson
Associate Program Officer
Board on Health Sciences Policy
Institute of Medicine

Lorraine M. Harkavy
Interdisciplinary Scientist
Biomedical Advanced Research
   and Development Authority
Office of the Assistant Secretary
   for Preparedness and Response

Robert Harrison
California Department of Public
   Health

Frank Hearl
Chief of Staff
National Institute for Occupational
   Safety and Health

David K. Henderson
Deputy Director for Clinical Care
Clinical Center, National Institutes
   of Health

Kent Hofacre
Manager
Battelle

David A. Hofmann
Hugh L. McColl Scholar in
   Leadership
University of North Carolina–
   Chapel Hill

Mylena Holguin
Senior Market Manager, Infection
   Control Apparel
Cardinal Health

James Hornstein
Vice President, Operations
Moldex Metric, Inc.

Christie Huff
Vice President, Marketing
Safe Life Corp.

Robert Irwin
Senior Advisor
CDC Influenza Coordination Unit

James James
Director, Center for Public Health
   Preparedness and Disaster
   Response
American Medical Association

John Jernigan
Centers for Disease Control and
   Prevention

Lieutenant Commander Tim Jirus
Office of the Chief of Naval
   Operations Safety Liaison

Melanie King
Centers for Disease Control and
   Prevention

William Kojola
Industrial Hygienist
Department of Occupational Safety
   and Health
AFL–CIO

David Kuhar
Centers for Disease Control and
   Prevention

Korlu Kuyon
Infection Preventionist
Department of Health and Mental
   Hygiene–Perkins Hospital

Kevin Landkrohn
Occupational Safety and Health
  Administration
U.S. Department of Labor

Elaine L. Larson
Professor of Pharmaceutical and
  Therapeutic Research
Columbia University School of
  Nursing

Marcelle Layton
Assistant Commissioner
Bureau of Communicable Disease
New York City Department of
  Health and Mental Hygiene

David LeGrande
Director, Occupational Safety and
  Health
Communications Workers of
  America

Donna Lemmert
Infection Prevention Coordinator
Baltimore Washington Medical
  Center

Andrew Levinson
Occupational Safety and Health
  Administration

Yolla Levitt
Marketing Manager
3M OHESD

William G. Lindsley
National Institute for Occupational
  Safety and Health

Cathy Liverman
Program Director
Institute of Medicine

Sarah Locke
Westat

Elizabeth Lockerby
Infection Preventionist
Walter Reed Army Medical Center

Atkinson Longmire
Occupational Safety and Health
  Administration

Darci MacNab
Global Strategic Marketing
  Manager
Kimberly-Clark

Zina Manji
Director, Regulatory Affairs
GlaxoSmithKline Consumer
  Healthcare

Tara Martin
GlaxoSmithKline

Brigette Master
3M

Nicole McCullough
Manager
Technical Services and Regulatory
  Affairs
3M

Allison McGeer
Director, Infection Control
Professor, Laboratory Medicine
  and Pathobiology
University of Toronto
Mount Sinai Hospital

Leslie McGorman
Program Officer of Public Health
Infectious Diseases Society of
  America

Ron McGraw
International Association of Fire
    Fighters Health and Safety
    Department

Kathleen McPhaul
Assistant Professor and Chair
Occupational Health Section,
    American Public Health
    Association (APHA)
University of Maryland and APHA

Maret Millard
Technical Service Specialist
3M Infection Prevention Division

Amanda Miller
Design Engineer
Avon Protection Systems

Donald Milton
Professor and Director
Maryland Institute for Applied
    Environmental Health
University of Maryland

Mary Mohyla
Director, Infection
    Control/Employee
    Health/Accreditation Services
Holy Cross Hospital

John A. Molinari
Director of Infection Control
The Dental Advisor

Sheila Murphey
Medical Officer
Food and Drug Administration

Elaine Namba
Research Scientist
Kimberly-Clark

Ingrid Nembhard
Assistant Professor
Division of Health Policy and
    Administration
Yale School of Public Health

Tom Nerad
Occupational Safety and Health
    Administration

William Newcomb
National Personal Protective
    Technology Laboratory
National Institute for Occupational
    Safety and Health

Mark Nicas
Adjunct Professor
University of California–Berkeley

Debra Novak
Senior Service Fellow
National Personal Protective
    Technology Laboratory
National Institute for Occupational
    Safety and Health

Anthony Oliver
Office of Emergency Medical
    Services

Carolyn Onye
Industrial Hygienist
U.S. Coast Guard

Amy Packman
Board Assistant
Institute of Medicine

Peter Palese
Professor and Chair
Department of Microbiology
Mount Sinai School of Medicine

Regina Pana-Cryan
Senior Scientist
National Institute for Occupational
Safety and Health

Kapil Panguluri
Food and Drug Administration

Stephanie Pasko
Senior Product Manager
Medline Industries, Inc.

Daniel R. Perez
Associate Professor
VA–MD Regional College of
Veterinary Medicine

Rogelio Pérez-Padilla
Director General
Instituto Nacional de Enfermedades
Respiratorias

Trish M. Perl
Director, Hospital Epidemiology
and Infection Control
Johns Hopkins University School
of Medicine

Jay Peterson
Industrial Hygienist
National Institutes of Health

Andrew M. Pope
Board Director
Institute of Medicine

David Prezant
Deputy Chief Medical Officer
New York City Fire Department

Lewis J. Radonovich
National Center for Occupational
Health and Infection Control
Veterans Health Administration
University of Florida

Virginia Rauer
Metropolitan Washington
Association of Occupational
Health Nurses, Inc.

Ann Reilly
Director, Employee Health
St. Joseph Medical Center

Raymond Roberge
National Personal Protective
Technology Laboratory
National Institute for Occupational
Safety and Health

Kathy Robinson
National Association of State EMS
Officials

Marc Roe
3M Company

M. E. Bonnie Rogers
Director, Occupational Safety and
Health
University of North Carolina
School of Public Health

Patricia Rosenbaum
Infection Preventionist Consultant
APIC

Cindy Rosenberger
Infection Preventionist
Kernan Orthopaedics and
Rehabilitation

Jack Ross
Hartford Hospital

Brenda Roup
Nurse Consultant, Infection
Prevention and Control
Maryland Department of Health
and Mental Hygiene

Kimberly Rumping
Program Specialist
Veterans Health Administration–
    National Center for Occupational
    Health and Infection Control

Bruce Russell
Preventive Medicine
    Administrative Officer
U.S. Army Medical Department
    Activity

Vicken Sarkissian
Sperian

Lisa Scheidelman
Infection Control Practitioner
St. Joseph Medical Center

Anita Schill
Associate Director for Science
National Institute for Occupational
    Safety and Health

Roslyne Schulman
Director, Policy Development
American Hospital Association

Renee Setteducato
Federation of Nurses/United
    Federation of Teachers

Ron Shaffer
Branch Chief
National Personal Protective
    Technology Laboratory
National Institute for Occupational
    Health and Safety

Kristina Sherry
Reporter/Editor
Inside Washington Publishers

Gilad Shoham
Medonyx, Inc., Canada

Rosemary Sokas
Director
Office of Occupational Medicine
Occupational Safety and Health
    Administration

Gwen Stewart
Infection Preventionist
Infection Control and
    Prevention/Employee Health
Sibley Memorial Hospital

Eileen Storey
Acting Chief, Surveillance Branch
Division of Respiratory Diseases
National Institute for Occupational
    Safety and Health

Jonathan Swerdlin
President
MM Herman and Associates, LLC

Linda Sylvester
Prince George's Hospital Center

Michael Tapper
Hospital Epidemiologist
Lenox Hill Hospital

Barbara Thieman
Laurel Regional Hospital

Greg Tilley
Principal Engineer
Avon Protection Systems

Lisa Tomlinson
Senior Director, Government
    Affairs
APIC

Jonathan Van-Tam
Professor of Health Protection
University of Nottingham

Joseph D. Wander
U.S. Air Force Research
    Laboratory

Richard P. Wenzel
Professor
Department of Internal Medicine
Virginia Commonwealth
    University School of Medicine

Katherine West
Infection Control/Emerging
    Concepts, Inc.

Gamunu Wijetunge
Office of EMS
National Highway Traffic Safety
    Administration
Department of Transportation

James Wilcox
Business Development Manager
Avon Protection Systems

Debbie Wilson
Team Leader
Employee Occupational Health
Inova Health System

Richard D. Wood
Manager, Global Industrial
    Hygiene Services
Air Products and Chemicals, Inc.

Annalee Yassi
Global Health Research Program
University of British Columbia

Theodore Yee
Medical Officer
Occupational Safety and Health
    Administration

Melanie T. Young
Policy and Strategic Initiatives
    Director
Society for Healthcare
    Epidemiology of America

C

Studies of the Clinical Effectiveness of Personal Protective Equipment During Outbreaks of Severe Acute Respiratory Syndrome and Respiratory Syncytial Virus

TABLE C-1 Studies of the Clinical Effectiveness of Personal Protective Equipment During Outbreaks of Severe Acute Respiratory Syndrome and Respiratory Syncytial Virus

Reference	Description	Results
Severe Acute Respiratory Syndrome (SARS)		
Seto et al., 2003	Case-control study in five Hong Kong hospitals of 13 SARS-infected staff and 241 non-infected staff	Odds ratio of staff with specific protection not getting infected: • Masks: OR= 13 (95% CI 3 to 60, $p = 0.0001$) • Gloves: OR = 2 (95% CI 0.6 to 7, $p = 0.364$) • Gowns: OR not calculated • Handwashing: OR = 5 (95% CI 1 to 19, $p = 0.047$)
Lau et al., 2004	Case-control study in Hong Kong of 72 hospital workers with SARS and 144 matched controls	• Risk of SARS infection in those reporting problems with mask fit: OR = 1.00 (95% CI 0.51 to 1.95, $p = 1.0000$) • Risk of SARS infection in those who had problems with fogging of goggles: OR = 0.61 (95% CI 0.31 to 1.17)

Continued

Reference	Description	Results
Loeb et al., 2004	Retrospective cohort study of 43 nurses working with SARS patients in Toronto critical care units	Risk of acquiring SARS based on use of PPE: • Gown: RR = 0.36 (95% CI 0.10 to 1.24, $p = 0.12$) • Gloves: RR = 0.45 (95% CI 0.14 to 1.46, $p = 0.22$) • N95 (respirator at least once) or surgical mask: RR = 0.23 (95% CI 0.07 to 0.78, $p = .02$) • N95: RR = 0.22 (95% CI 0.05 to 0.93, $p = 0.06$) • Surgical mask:[a] RR = 0.45 (95% CI 0.07 to 2.71, $p = 0.56$) • N95 vs. surgical mask:[b] RR = 0.50 (95% CI 0.06 to 4.23, $p = 0.51$)
Teleman et al., 2004	Case-control study in Singapore of 36 healthcare workers with probable SARS and 50 healthcare workers in the same ward with history of exposure	Adjusted odds ratio (multivariate analysis) associated with transmission of SARS: • Wearing of N95 mask: 0.1 (95% CI 0.02 to 0.9, $p = 0.04$) • Wearing of gloves: 1.5 (95% CI 0.3 to 7.2, $p = 0.6$) • Wearing of gowns: 0.5 (95% CI 0.4 to 6.9, $p = 0.6$) • Handwashing after each patient: 0.07 (95% CI 0.008 to 0.7, $p = 0.02$)

Respiratory Syncytial Virus (RSV)

Reference	Description	Results

Hall and Douglas, 1981	Comparison of use and nonuse of gowns and masks by staff members on a pediatric ward with children < 3 years old	• Proportion of infants acquiring RSV:
		  o When masks and gowns were used by staff: 32%
		  o When masks and gowns were not used by staff: 41%
		• Proportion of staff acquiring RSV:
		  o During the time masks and gowns were used by staff: 33%
		  o During the time masks and gowns were not used by staff: 42%
		• Measurable benefit not found in controlling spread of RSV

Murphy et al., 1981	Prospective study of use and nonuse of masks and gowns by staff members caring for infants with respiratory disease	• Number of RSV or other respiratory infections did not differ significantly between the two groups of staff (handwashing only; and handwashing, gowning, and masking)

Reference	Description	Results
Gala et al., 1986	Comparison of use and nonuse of eye–nose goggles by staff members on an infant ward	• Frequency of RSV infection in hospital personnel: ○ Three weeks during goggle use: 8% ($p = 0.003$) ○ Three weeks with no goggle use: 34% ($p = 0.003$)
Agah et al., 1987	Comparison of use and nonuse of mask or goggles by staff members caring for children with RSV infections on a pediatric inpatient service	• RSV illness rate in healthcare workers caring for children with RSV infections: ○ Wore masks or goggles: 5% ($p < 0.01$ compared to no masks or goggles category) ○ Did not wear masks or goggles: 61%
Madge et al., 1992	Prospective study of four infection control strategies in preventing RSV in four pediatric wards	• Combination of cohort nursing with use of gowns and gloves significantly reduced RSV infection • Use of gowns and gloves alone did not result in a significant reduction of infection
Langley et al., 1997	Prospective cohort study comparing isolation policies and RSV infections in pediatric patients in nine hospitals	• Various combinations of requirements for use of gowns, gloves, and masks did not result in decreased nosocomial rates in patients; gowning for any entry to the patient's room was associated with increased risk of RSV transmission

NOTE: CI = confidence interval; OR = odds ratio; RR = relative risk.
The terms (*masks*, *surgical masks*, and *respirators*) used in this table are those used by the investigators or authors of the cited journal article or report. In some cases, it is not possible to determine whether the authors' use of the term *masks* refers to medical masks, respirators, or both.
[a] Comparator is use of no mask.
[b] Consistent use of N95 versus consistent use of surgical mask.
SOURCE: IOM (2008).

REFERENCES

Agah, R., J. D. Cherry, A. J. Garakian, and M. Chapin. 1987. Respiratory syncytial virus (RSV) infection rate in personnel caring for children with RSV infections. Routine isolation procedure vs routine procedure supplemented by use of masks and goggles. *American Journal of Diseases of Children* 141(6):695-697.

Gala, C. L., C. B. Hall, K. C. Schnabel, P. H. Pincus, P. Blossom, S. W. Hildreth, R. F. Betts, and R. G. Douglas, Jr. 1986. The use of eye-nose goggles to control nosocomial respiratory syncytial virus infection. *Journal of the American Medical Association* 256(19):2706-2708.

Hall, C. B., and R. G. Douglas, Jr. 1981. Nosocomial respiratory syncytial viral infections. Should gowns and masks be used? *American Journal of Diseases of Children* 135(6):512-515.

IOM (Institute of Medicine). 2008. *Preparing for an influenza pandemic: Personal protective equipment for healthcare workers.* Washington, DC: The National Academies Press.

Langley, J. M., J. C. LeBlanc, E. E. Wang, B. J. Law, N. E. MacDonald, I. Mitchell, D. Stephens, J. McDonald, F. D. Boucher, and S. Dobson. 1997. Nosocomial respiratory syncytial virus infection in Canadian pediatric hospitals: A Pediatric Investigators Collaborative Network on Infections in Canada Study. *Pediatrics* 100(6):943-946.

Lau, J. T., K. S. Fung, T. W. Wong, J. H. Kim, E. Wong, S. Chung, D. Ho, L. Y. Chan, S. F. Lui, and A. Cheng. 2004. SARS transmission among hospital workers in Hong Kong. *Emerging Infectious Diseases* 10(2):280-286.

Loeb, M., A. McGeer, B. Henry, M. Ofner, D. Rose, T. Hlywka, J. Levie, J. McQueen, S. Smith, L. Moss, A. Smith, K. Green, and S. D. Walter. 2004. SARS among critical care nurses, Toronto. *Emerging Infectious Diseases* 10(2):251-255.

Madge, P., J. Y. Paton, J. H. McColl, and P. L. Mackie. 1992. Prospective controlled study of four infection-control procedures to prevent nosocomial infection with respiratory syncytial virus. *Lancet* 340(8827):1079-1083.

Murphy, D., J. K. Todd, R. K. Chao, I. Orr, and K. McIntosh. 1981. The use of gowns and masks to control respiratory illness in pediatric hospital personnel. *Journal of Pediatrics* 99(5):746-750.

Seto, W. H., D. Tsang, R. W. Yung, T. Y. Ching, T. K. Ng, M. Ho, L. M. Ho, and J. S. Peiris. 2003. Effectiveness of precautions against droplets and contact in prevention of nosocomial transmission of severe acute respiratory syndrome (SARS). *Lancet* 361(9368):1519-1520.

Teleman, M. D., I. C. Boudville, B. H. Heng, D. Zhu, and Y. S. Leo. 2004. Factors associated with transmission of severe acute respiratory syndrome among health-care workers in Singapore. *Epidemiology and Infection* 132(5):797-803.

D

Examples of Relevant Voluntary Consensus Standards

ASTM International standards are used extensively by the Food and Drug Administration (FDA) for 510k submissions of personal protective equipment (PPE). Examples of standards relevant to PPE used by healthcare workers include the following:

D3577 Specification for Rubber Surgical Gloves
D3578 Specification for Rubber Examination Gloves
D5151 Test Method for Detection of Holes in Medical Gloves
D5250 Specification for Poly(Vinyl Chloride) Gloves for Medical Application
D6124 Test Method for Residual Powder on Medical Gloves
D6319 Specification for Nitrile Examination Gloves for Medical Application
D6499 Test Method for the Immunological Measurement of Antigenic Protein in Natural Rubber and Its Products
D6977 Specification for Polychloroprene Examination Gloves for Medical Application
F1671 Test Method for Resistance of Materials Used in Protective Clothing to Penetration by Blood-Borne Pathogens Using Phi-X174 Bacteriophage Penetration as a Test System
F1862 Standard Test Method for Resistance of Medical Face Masks to Penetration by Synthetic Blood (Horizontal Projection of Fixed Volume at a Known Velocity)
F2101 Standard Test Method for Evaluating the Bacterial Filtration Efficiency of Surgical Masks Using a Biological Aerosol of Staphylococcus aureus
F2407 Standard Specification for Surgical Gowns Intended for Use in Healthcare Facilities

American National Standards Institute (ANSI)

ANSI has standards that include guidance to employers for the practice of respiratory protection, but not the devices themselves. These include the following:

Z88.2   Practices for Respiratory Protection
Z88.6   Medical Qualifications of Respirator Wearers
Z88.10 Fit-Test Requirements for Respiratory Protection

The Occupational Safety and Health Administration has incorporated the following ANSI standard into its eye and face protection standard (Code of Federal Regulations 1919.133):

Z87.1   Standard Practice for Occupational and Educational Eye and Face Protection

Association for Advancement of Medical Instrumentation (AAMI)

AAMI has a standard for fluid resistance of gowns worn by healthcare workers. Minimum performance levels ranging from 1 (least protective) to 4 (most protective) have been determined. These levels apply to the product's Critical Zone, including seams, but excluding cuffs, hems, and bindings.

National Fire Protection Association (NFPA) Standards

The FDA includes the following NFPA standard into its requirements for masks and respirators:

702   Standard for Classification of Flammability of Wearing Apparel

Another example of a relevant NFPA standard includes

NFPA1999   Standard on Protective Clothing for Emergency Medical Operations

E

Committee Biographies

Elaine L. Larson, R.N., Ph.D., FAAN, CIC (*Chair*), is associate dean for research and professor of pharmaceutical and therapeutic research, Columbia University School of Nursing, and professor of epidemiology, Columbia University Mailman School of Public Health. She is a former dean of Georgetown University School of Nursing. Dr. Larson has been a member of the Board of Directors, National Foundation for Infectious Diseases, and the Report Review Committee, National Academy of Sciences. She is the director of the Center for Interdisciplinary Research to Prevent Antimicrobial Resistance at Columbia University and has been editor of the *American Journal of Infection Control* since 1994. She has published more than 200 journal articles, 4 books, and a number of book chapters in the areas of infection prevention, epidemiology, and clinical research.

Gloria Addo-Ayensu, M.D., M.P.H., is the director of health for Fairfax County, VA. In this capacity she provides overall direction for public health programs in the county, including emergency preparedness. She has led Fairfax County's comprehensive pandemic influenza preparedness efforts and engaged a wide range of community stakeholders in the process. As past chair of the Metropolitan Washington Council of Governments Health Officials Committee, she facilitated initial coordination of the National Capital Region's pandemic planning in 2006. Dr. Addo-Ayensu is interested in international health and has served as a consultant to research and public health programs in Ghana.

Allison E. Aiello, Ph.D., is the John G. Searle Assistant Professor of Public Health at the University of Michigan School of Public Health in the

Department of Epidemiology. Dr. Aiello held a Robert Wood Johnson Foundation Health and Society Scholars Fellowship at the University of Michigan and an Emerging Infectious Diseases Fellowship at the Centers for Disease Control and Prevention (CDC). Dr. Aiello's research focuses on the use of non-pharmaceutical interventions, including masks and hand hygiene interventions, for mitigating influenza transmission. She also investigates socioeconomic and race/ethnic disparities in infectious diseases, the relationship between infection and chronic diseases, and the emergence of antimicrobial resistance in the community setting. Her work on these topics has been presented at numerous national and international conferences and published in peer-reviewed journals, including *Lancet Infectious Diseases, Emerging Infectious Diseases, American Journal of Public Health, Journal of Infectious Diseases, Clinical Infectious Diseases*, and the *American Journal of Epidemiology*. Dr. Aiello is on the editorial board of the *American Journal of Infection Control*, associate editor of *BMC Public Health*, and an invited member of the American College of Epidemiology Minority Affairs Committee. She received her Ph.D. in epidemiology from Columbia University's Mailman School of Public Health, where she held a National Institute of Allergy and Infectious Diseases training fellowship and was the recipient of the Ana C. Gelman Award for outstanding achievement and promise in the field of epidemiology.

Howard J. Cohen, Ph.D., M.P.H., CIH, is professor emeritus (formerly professor and chair of the Occupational Safety and Health Department) at the University of New Haven. He is an associate (adjunct) professor at Yale University's Department of Occupational and Environmental Medicine. He formerly was the manager of industrial hygiene at the Olin Corporation and editor in chief of the *American Industrial Hygiene Association Journal*. He is certified in the comprehensive practice of industrial hygiene by the American Board of Industrial Hygiene. Dr. Cohen is the former chair of the American National Standards Institute Z88.2 committee on respiratory protection and a current member of the editorial board of the *Journal of Occupational and Environmental Hygiene*. He is the past chair of the American Industrial Hygiene Association's (AIHA's) respiratory protection committee, a past president of the Connecticut River Valley Chapter of the AIHA, and a past officer and treasurer of the American Board of Industrial Hygiene. Dr. Cohen served on the Institute of Medicine (IOM) Committee on Personal Protective Equipment for Healthcare Workers During an Influenza Pandemic and on the IOM

Standing Committee on Personal Protective Equipment for Workplace Safety and Health. He is currently working as a consultant to the Veterans Administration's North Florida/South Georgia Center for Occupational Safety and Infectious Disease (on the Advisory Board and assisting on an upcoming clinical study of influenza). Dr. Cohen is also a consultant to a pharmaceutical company that has developed the first antiviral N95 surgical respirator to be certified by the Food and Drug Administration (FDA) and National Institute for Occupational Safety and Health (NIOSH). He is a graduate of Boston University, where he received a B.A. in biology. Dr. Cohen received his M.P.H. and Ph.D. in industrial health from the University of Michigan.

Robert Cohen, M.D., FCCP, is chair of the Division of Pulmonary and Critical Care Medicine for the Cook County Health and Hospitals System and chair of pulmonary and critical care medicine at the John H. Stroger, Jr., Hospital of Cook County, IL. His early research focused on the resurgent epidemic of tuberculosis in the City of Chicago and at Cook County Hospital. Dr. Cohen has worked closely with patients suffering from chronic obstructive pulmonary disease (COPD), and he founded Cook County Hospital's pulmonary rehabilitation program. He has worked as the medical director of the Black Lung Clinics at Cook County Hospital and as medical director of the federally funded Black Lung Clinics Program, a program dedicated to the care of coal miners throughout the United States. He has worked closely with the American Lung Association of Metropolitan Chicago and is a member of the American Lung Association's COPD task force, currently serving as the medical director of the Community Spirometry Initiative. He is a recipient of its Public Health Service Award in 2006 and Outstanding Clinician Award in 2007. Dr. Cohen's work on respiratory disease in coal mining populations has involved consulting in areas of mining-related health issues for federal agencies, including the U.S. Agency for International Development (USAID), CDC, and NIOSH. He has recently served as a member of the Mine Safety Research Advisory Committee. In addition, he has provided expert consultation on occupational lung disease to clinics supported by USAID in Donetsk, Ukraine. Dr. Cohen graduated from Northwestern University's Honors Program in Medical Education in 1981. He did his internship and residency at Cook County Hospital, as well as subspecialty training in pulmonary medicine and critical care.

Karen Coyne, Ph.D., is research general engineer at the U.S. Army Edgewood Chemical Biological Center (ECBC). Dr. Coyne has 8 years of experience in respiratory protection research and testing at the U.S. Army ECBC. Her specific areas of expertise are in testing and modeling the physiological impact of wearing respiratory protection and in developing novel test systems. Prior to this, she spent 7 years at the University of Maryland–College Park (UMCP), conducting respiratory protection research and developing data collection and instrumentation systems for assessing the impact of protective equipment on respiration, vision, communications, and work performance. Dr. Coyne has authored or coauthored 20 journal publications, 8 technical reports, and 18 platform (2 international) and 6 poster conference presentations, has given 5 university guest lectures, and is coinventor on a patent. She taught a physiological modeling course at UMCP for 3 years. She served as a member of the Project B.R.E.A.T.H.E. working group. Dr. Coyne won the John White Best Paper Award in respiratory protection from the *Journal of Occupational and Environmental Hygiene* for 2000 and 2006 and the Michigan Industrial Hygiene Society Best Paper award in 1998. She received her Ph.D. in biological resources engineering from UMCP.

David M. DeJoy, Ph.D., is professor of health promotion and behavior and director of the Workplace Health Group in the College of Public Health at the University of Georgia. Dr. DeJoy has 30 years of experience in workplace safety and health as a researcher, instructor, and consultant. His areas of research include safety climate/culture, work organization, safe work practices, risk communication, and theory-based intervention design/intervention effectiveness. He has published approximately 120 scientific articles and book chapters and presented more than 200 papers at scientific and professional meetings. He currently serves on the editorial boards of *Safety Science, Journal of Safety Research,* and *Journal of Occupational Health Psychology.* Extramural funding for his research has come from CDC, the National Institutes of Health (NIH), and NIOSH. Dr. DeJoy has served on numerous expert panels, review committees, and advisory panels at the national and international levels.

Ken Gall, Ph.D., is a professor in the School of Materials Science and Engineering and Mechanical Engineering at the Georgia Institute of Technology. Before joining Georgia Tech in 2005, he was an associate professor of mechanical engineering at the University of Colorado at Boulder and a post-doc at Sandia National Laboratories. Dr. Gall's research combines polymer chemistry, materials science, bioengineering, and mechanical engineering in order to synthesize and characterize new materials for use in emerging technologies. His specific interests include metallic and polymer biomaterials, mechanically active materials, and nanometer scale materials and characterization. He has published more than 130 journal articles, which have been cited more than 2,200 times, and he has given approximately 200 professional talks. He has provided extensive consulting on materials and engineering for law firms, industry, national labs, and the U.S. military. His research on shape memory alloys and polymers was the basis for founding MedShape Solutions, a company developing shape memory material-based orthopedic devices. He received his B.S., M.S., and Ph.D. in mechanical engineering from the University of Illinois.

William H. Kojola, M.S., is the industrial hygienist for the American Federation of Labor and Congress of Industrial Organizations' (AFL–CIO's) Department of Occupational Health and Safety. His experience in health and safety spans more than 30 years. During that time, Mr. Kojola has been the director of the Occupational Safety and Health Division of the Laborers Health and Safety Fund of North America, an occupational safety and health specialist for the International Brotherhood of Boilermakers, and director of safety and health for the United Cement, Lime, Gypsum and Allied Workers International Union. Prior to this, he was a health research scientist at the University of Illinois School of Public Health, studying the human health effects of air and water pollutants. With the AFL–CIO, Mr. Kojola is responsible for developing strategies for securing new safety and health protections through federal and state regulations, coordinating with affiliates on and leading a unified labor response to proposed Occupational Safety and Health Administration (OSHA) regulations, and representing the AFL–CIO before government regulatory agencies, on federal advisory committees, and in consensus standard-setting efforts. He also works with affiliate unions to address emerging workplace hazards and issues. Mr. Kojola holds a B.S. in biology and an M.S. in genetics from the University of Minnesota, and studied toxicology and industrial hygiene at the University of Illinois School of Public Health.

Allison McGeer, M.D., is a professor in the Departments of Laboratory Medicine and Pathobiology and at the Dalla Lana School of Public Health at the University of Toronto. In addition to her positions as microbiologist and director of infection control at Mount Sinai Hospital, Toronto, Dr. McGeer is an infection control consultant to the Baycrest Centre for Geriatric Care. She currently serves on Canada's National Advisory Committee on Immunization and on the infection control sub-committee of the Ontario Provincial Infectious Diseases Advisory Com-mittee. She is a member of several local, provincial, and national pan-demic influenza committees. She is an expert reviewer for many research funding agencies, including the Canadian Institute of Health Research and U.S. NIH, and has served on the editorial boards of several journals, including the *Canadian Medical Association Journal* and *Infection Con-trol and Hospital Epidemiology*. She returned to Mount Sinai Hospital in 1989 as a microbiologist and director of infection control. Her major re-search interests are in the prevention of infection in hospitals and nursing homes, and the use of surveillance to advance the prevention, diagnosis, and treatment of infectious diseases. She is the principal investigator of the Toronto Invasive Bacterial Diseases Network and the Ontario Group A Streptococcal Study, two collaborative surveillance networks studying the epidemiology of severe community-acquired infections. Dr. McGeer served on the Council of Canadian Academies expert panel on influenza transmission and the role of personal protective equipment, and on the IOM Committee on the Development of Reusable Facemasks for Use During an Influenza Pandemic. Dr. McGeer completed an undergraduate and master's degree in biochemistry and her M.D. at the University of Toronto. She specialized in internal medicine and infectious diseases, followed by a fellowship in hospital epidemiology at Yale New Haven Hospital.

Peter Palese, Ph.D., is a professor of microbiology and chair of the De-partment of Microbiology at the Mount Sinai School of Medicine in New York. His scientific publications include research on the replication of ribonucleic acid (RNA)–containing viruses, with a special emphasis on influenza viruses, which are negative-strand RNA viruses. Specifically, he established the first genetic maps for influenza A, B, and C viruses; identified the function of several viral genes; and defined the mechanism of neuraminidase inhibitors (which are now FDA-approved antivirals). Dr. Palese also pioneered the field of reverse genetics for negative-strand RNA viruses, which allows the introduction of site-specific mutations into the genomes of these viruses. This technique is crucial for the study of the structure/function relationships of viral genes, for investigation of viral pathogenicity, and for development and manufacture of influenza virus vaccines. In addition, an improvement of the technique has been used effectively to reconstruct and study the pathogenicity of the highly virulent but extinct 1918 pandemic influenza virus. His recent work in collaboration with Dr. Adolfo Garcia-Sastre has revealed that most negative-strand RNA viruses possess proteins with interferon antagonist activity, enabling them to counteract the antiviral response of the infected host. Dr. Palese was elected to the National Academy of Sciences in 2000 for his seminal studies on influenza viruses. He serves on the editorial board for the *Proceedings of the National Academy of Sciences* and as an editor for the *Journal of Virology*. Dr. Palese was president of the Harvey Society in 2004 and is a past president of the American Society for Virology.

David Prezant, M.D., is the chief medical officer and special advisor to the fire commissioner for health policy, fire department of the City of New York (FDNY). He is also a professor of medicine in the Pulmonary Division at Albert Einstein College of Medicine. Dr. Prezant is board certified in internal medicine, pulmonary medicine, and critical care medicine. He is a member of the John P. Redmond International Association of Fire Fighters Medical Advisory Board and represents FDNY as a member of the technical committee for the Fire Service Joint Labor Management Wellness/Fitness Initiative. Dr. Prezant is the author of numerous peer-reviewed articles on the health and safety of firefighters, thermal protective equipment to reduce burn injuries and improve exercise performance for firefighters, and recently the effect of World Trade Center exposures on respiratory health of firefighters and emergency medical services personnel. Dr. Prezant serves on the IOM Standing Committee on Personal Protective Equipment for Workplace Safety and Health. He was a member of the IOM Committee on Personal Protective Equipment for Healthcare Workers During an Influenza Pandemic and the IOM Committee to Review the NIOSH Personal Protective Technology Program. He received his B.S. from Columbia College and his M.D. from the Albert Einstein College of Medicine.

M. E. Bonnie Rogers, Dr.P.H., M.P.H., COHN-S, LNNC, FAAN, is an associate professor of nursing and public health and director of the North Carolina Occupational Safety and Health Education and Research Center and the Occupational Health Nursing Program at the University of North Carolina, School of Public Health, Chapel Hill. Dr. Rogers was a visiting scholar at the Hasting Center in New York and is an ethics consultant. She is certified in occupational health nursing and as a legal nurse consultant. Dr. Rogers is a fellow in the American Academy of Nursing and the American Association of Occupational Health Nurses. Dr. Rogers serves as chair of the NIOSH National Occupational Research Agenda Liaison Committee. She has served on numerous IOM committees, including the Committee on Personal Protective Equipment for Healthcare Workers During an Influenza Pandemic and on the IOM Standing Committee on Personal Protective Equipment for Workplace Safety and Health. Dr. Rogers chaired the recent fast-track IOM study, Respiratory Protection for Healthcare Workers in the Workplace Against Novel H1N1 Influenza A. She has served in leadership positions for occupational health professional societies and is past president of the American Association of Occupational Health Nurses and the Association of Occupational and Environmental Clinics. Dr. Rogers is currently vice president of the International Commission on Occupational Health. She received her diploma in nursing from the Washington Hospital Center School of Nursing, Washington, DC; her baccalaureate in nursing from George Mason University, School of Nursing, Fairfax, VA; and her M.P.H. and Dr.P.H. from the Johns Hopkins University School of Hygiene and Public Health.

Richard P. Wenzel, M.D., M.Sc., is professor and former chair of the Department of Internal Medicine at the Medical College of Virginia (MCV), Virginia Commonwealth University (1995–2009). From 2003 to 2008, he was president of MCV Physicians, the clinical practice plan for more than 600 physicians, and senior associate dean for clinical affairs. Dr. Wenzel's research has focused on the prevention and control of hospital-acquired infections, especially bloodstream infections and sepsis. He is a nationally recognized expert on antibiotic resistance and its impact. He has served on the editorial board of *New England Journal of Medicine* and, in 2001, became the journal's first editor at large, a position he still holds. Dr. Wenzel has authored more than 500 publications and is editor of 6 textbooks, including *A Guide for Infection Control in the Hospital*, which has been translated into 8 languages for free distribution to healthcare workers in developing countries. His popular book, *Stalking Microbes*, was published in summer 2005. A medical thriller, *Labyrinth of Terror*, was released in 2010. Dr. Wenzel is a member of the American Society of Clinical Investigation and the Association of American Physicians and a charter member of the Surgical Infections Society. He is also former president of the Society of Healthcare Epidemiology of America.

From 2006 to 2008, Dr. Wenzel was president of the International Socie-ty for Infectious Diseases. He has received numerous awards for research and teaching, including the Humboldt Research Award for Senior U.S. Scientists, a Senior International Fellowship Fogarty Award from the National Institutes of Health, and the Bruce Award from the American College of Physicians–American Society of Internal Medicine.